T0234822

The Wills Eye
STRABISMUS
SURGERY
Handbook

The Wills Eye
STRABISMUS
SURGERY
Handbook

Editors

Leonard B. Nelson, MD, MBA

Director of the Strabismus Center

*Co-Director of the Department of Pediatric Ophthalmology
and Ocular Genetics*

Wills Eye Hospital

Philadelphia, Pennsylvania

Alex V. Levin, MD, MHSc, FRCSC

Chief, Pediatric Ophthalmology and Ocular Genetics

*Robison D. Harley, MD Endowed Chair in Pediatric Ophthalmology
and Ocular Genetics*

Wills Eye Hospital

Philadelphia, Pennsylvania

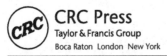

CRC Press
Taylor & Francis Group
Boca Raton London New York

CRC Press is an imprint of the
Taylor & Francis Group, an **informa** business

First published 2015 by SLACK Incorporated

Published 2024 by CRC Press
2385 NW Executive Center Drive, Suite 320, Boca Raton FL 33431

and by CRC Press
4 Park Square, Milton Park, Abingdon, Oxon, OX14 4RN

CRC Press is an imprint of Taylor & Francis Group, LLC

Library of Congress Cataloging-in-Publication Data

The Wills Eye strabismus surgery handbook / editors, Leonard B. Nelson, Alex V. Levin.
    p. ; cm.
Strabismus surgery handbook
Includes bibliographical references and index.
ISBN 978-1-61711-968-2 (alk. paper)
I. Nelson, Leonard B. editor. II. Levin, Alex V., editor. III. Wills Eye Hospital (Philadelphia, Pa.), issuing body. IV. Title: Strabismus surgery handbook.
    [DNLM: 1. Strabismus--surgery--Handbooks. 2. Ophthalmologic Surgical Procedures--methods--Handbooks. WW 39]
    RE771
    617.7'62--dc23

                                2015003427

ISBN: 9781617119682 (pbk)
ISBN: 9781003526940 (ebk)

DOI: 10.1201/9781003526940

CONTENTS

Acknowledgments .... *vii*

About the Editors .... *ix*

Contributing Authors .... *xi*

Preface .... *xiii*

Foreword by Stephen P. Kraft, MD, FRCSC. .... *xv*

Abbreviations .... *xvii*

Chapter 1   Approach to Strabismus Surgery Decision Making 1
             Leonard B. Nelson, MD, MBA

Chapter 2   Esotropia. 7
             Scott Olitsky, MD

Chapter 3   Exotropia 15
             Daniel T. Weaver, MD

Chapter 4   Dissociated Vertical Deviation 25
             Sepideh Tara Rousta, MD

Chapter 5   Cranial Nerve Palsies 33
             Mary O'Hara, MD

Chapter 6   Strabismus Syndromes 45
             Mark A. Steele, MD

Chapter 7   Strabismus in Systemic Disease 57
             Miles J. Burke, MD

Chapter 8   Other Complex Strabismus Cases 75
             Kammi Gunton, MD

Chapter 9   Reoperations 87
             Rudolph S. Wagner, MD

Chapter 10   Nystagmus 99
             Leonard B. Nelson, MD, MBA

Financial Disclosures. 105

Index 107

ACKNOWLEDGMENTS

With the blessing of our colleagues from The Hospital for Sick Children, Drs. Steve Kraft, Ray Buncic, and David Smith, and with enormous gratitude to their contributions and guidance that allowed so many to learn strabismus (including Dr. Levin!) and help our fellows become strabismologists year after year, we decided to bring Strabismus Workbook to life. Thanks also to those fellows year after year who helped us think about these problems and continue to give us the privilege of teaching them.

All of this would not have been possible without the patients who help us become better doctors and surgeons and our families who have supported us through the process.

Alex V. Levin, MD, MHSc, FRCSC
Leonard B. Nelson, MD

ABOUT THE EDITORS

Leonard B. Nelson, MD, MBA, received a BA in biology from Columbia University and his MD from Harvard Medical School. Following a surgical internship at Harvard, he completed his ophthalmology residency at New York University Bellevue Hospital Medical Center. He went on to complete a 1-year fellowship in Pediatric Ophthalmology at the Children's National Medical Center and a 1-year fellowship in ocular genetics at the Wilmer Institute. He obtained his MBA at St. Joseph's University. Dr. Nelson is the Director of the Strabismus Center and the Co-Director of the Pediatric Ophthalmology and Ocular Genetics Department at Wills Eye Hospital.

Alex V. Levin, M.D., MHSc, FAAP, FAAO, FRCSC, was a child abuse pediatrician following completion of a pediatric residency at the Children's Hospital of Philadelphia. He then completed an ophthalmology residency at Wills Eye Hospital in Philadelphia, followed by a pediatric ophthalmology fellowship at The Hospital for Sick Children in Toronto, where he returned to become a professor in the Departments of Pediatrics, Genetics and Ophthalmology and Vision Sciences at the University of Toronto while working as a staff ophthalmologist at The Hospital for Sick Children for over 16 years. There he was the Fellowship Director for 15 years and, with his colleagues, started the Strabismus Nights, which became the inspiration for this book. He is one of fewer than 10 double-boarded pediatrician-pediatric ophthalmologists in the world. In 2001, he obtained his master's degree in bioethics. In 2008, he returned to Wills Eye Hospital as the Chief of Pediatric Ophthalmology and Ocular Genetics.

CONTRIBUTING AUTHORS

Miles J. Burke, MD (Chapter 7)
Private Practice
Cincinnati, Ohio

Kammi Gunton, MD (Chapter 8)
Assistant Surgeon, Wills Eye Hospital
Assistant Professor of Ophthalmology, Thomas Jefferson University Hospital
Philadelphia, Pennsylvania

Stephen P. Kraft, MD, FRCSC (Foreword)
Professor, Department of Ophthalmology and Vision Sciences, Faculty of
    Medicine, University of Toronto
Staff Ophthalmologist, Department of Ophthalmology and Vision Sciences,
    The Hospital for Sick Children
Toronto, Canada

Mary O'Hara, MD (Chapter 5)
Professor, Departments of Ophthalmology & Pediatrics
University of California, Davis
Sacramento, California

Scott Olitsky, MD (Chapter 2)
Section Chief of Ophthalmology, Children's Mercy Hospital
Professor of Ophthalmology, University of Missouri–Kansas City School of
    Medicine
Associate Clinical Professor of Ophthalmology, University of Kansas School
    of Medicine
Kansas City, Missouri

Sepideh Tara Rousta, MD (Chapter 4)
Clinical Assistant Professor of Ophthalmology, Robert Wood Johnson
    University Hospital and Saint Peter's University Hospital
New Brunswick, New Jersey
Clinical Instructor, Wills Eye Hospital
Philadelphia, Pennsylvania

Mark A. Steele, MD (Chapter 6)
Clinical Associate Professor of Ophthalmology
Chief, Pediatric Ophthalmology and Strabismus Surgery
New York University–Langone Medical Center
New York, New York

Rudolph S. Wagner, MD (Chapter 9)
Clinical Professor of Ophthalmology
Director of Pediatric Ophthalmology
Rutgers–New Jersey Medical School
Newark, New Jersey

Daniel T. Weaver, MD (Chapter 3)
Adjunct Professor of Clinical Medicine, Rocky Mountain College
Pediatric Ophthalmologist, Billings Clinic
Billings, Montana

PREFACE

The Wills Eye Strabismus Surgery Handbook is designed to be an education manual for residents and pediatric ophthalmology fellows focused on developing surgical plans for strabismus patients. This book is also intended for comprehensive ophthalmologists and strabismus subspecialists. Each chapter begins with an introduction into the decision-making process of the author for the specific strabismus condition. This is followed by the surgical plans selected by three expert Wills Eye Strabismus Center strabismologists for the presented cases. Finally, the chapter author briefly reviews the basic concepts in developing a diagnosis and treatment plan while bringing together the varied opinions offered by the strabismologists to put them in context.

Obtaining continuity of care for strabismus patients is one of the challenges in residency and fellowship education. Although residents and fellows examine patients in the clinics, they are rarely involved in the surgery on the specific patients they see, and even less often get to follow the progress of these patients postoperatively. This makes the development of a treatment plan particularly challenging. In addition, trainees are often moving the muscles as selected by the attending. This book will give trainees the opportunity to develop the skills for surgical planning. We hope that it will also be an excellent aid for written and oral board preparation.

We are hoping that you, the reader, will use this book as more than a reference. Remember, there is no right answer for many strabismus challenges, but there are principles and considerations that can guide you to a better answer for your patient. Writing this book helped us appreciate the wide range of surgical practice, and we know you will come to appreciate this as well. We wish all of you success in the complicated world of strabismus surgery.

Leonard B. Nelson, MD, MBA
Alex V. Levin, MD, MHSc, FRCSC
Wills Eye Hospital
Philadelphia, Pennsylvania

FOREWORD

"Well, it depends…"

This is a phrase that is familiar to all 140 pediatric ophthalmology fellows I have helped train at Toronto's Hospital for Sick Children since 1984. They come armed with a wide range of knowledge and surgical experience in strabismus. Most of them have arrived with good grounding in the basics of the field, and the majority have the ability to formulate appropriate surgical plans for straightforward cases, especially comitant esotropias and exotropias.

Even within these seemingly routine cases, there lurk alternative approaches to diagnosis and surgical treatment. If a single strabismus label has different facets, it can lead to a variety of valid strategies for correcting it. As well, experienced strabismus surgeons can have alternative, and even opposing, proposals for the optimal surgical plan when considering the same case.

For example, when a fellow asks about my surgical approach for a case of comitant esotropia of 40 prism diopters, my answer is always: "Well, it depends…" Are we discussing an infantile esotropia or a partially accommodative esotropia? If it is an infantile esotropia, is the patient 6 months old or 10 years old? If a refractive correction is worn, is it a very high plus correction? Is there concurrent manifest latent nystagmus (also termed fusion maldevelopment nystagmus syndrome) or not? And so on. I have the same response for almost all other situations that trainees throw at us. One has to analyze many aspects of the problem to give a cogent answer.

A seemingly simple question can lead trainees, and attendings, down a garden of many possible paths, each with differing outcomes in terms of decision making. This is the joy of strabismus—a challenging compendium of puzzles with many facets that naturally lead to rich discussions.

To foster the analytical thought process that underlies so much of our specialty, Dr. Alex Levin spearheaded a forward-thinking initiative when he served as our Pediatric Ophthalmology Fellowship Director in Toronto. He worked with me and Drs. David Smith and Ray Buncic to establish bi-monthly Strabismus Nights. The four of us created a series of problem sets, akin to the worksheets that we recall from our undergraduate days in chemistry, mathematics, and physics. We created six documents under different themes, all involving surgical decision making, which increased in difficulty as the yearly cycle progressed. Each list had up to 20 related problems for the fellows to review, and we asked them to come prepared to discuss possible solutions on the assigned evening.

These evening sessions were initiated in the 1990s, and they continue at our hospital to this day. At these sessions, the trainees receive the undivided attention of the attending strabismus surgeons, as well as a great meal! A session can easily run for three hours, but the time always flies. During the course of the year, the attendings watch our trainees hone their diagnostic and thinking skills in analyzing these problems, whether simple or complex. And we also see firsthand how they apply this thinking to cases in the clinics, with increasing confidence and depth of discussion around case management. By the end of the year, most of them have developed an advanced analytical approach to strabismus with which they can tackle the great variety of cases they will face as they begin their careers in the strabismus world.

Drs. Nelson and Levin, along with their colleagues at Wills Eye and their former fellows, have undertaken a wonderful initiative by enlarging and publishing the problem sets we created back then and producing this workbook of solutions. The range of answers provided by this team of experts will give any trainee learning strabismus, as well as the budding strabismologist, a sampling of the complex thinking that underlies successful surgical planning in this field.

It underscores the fact that there is not necessarily one approach to solving a strabismus problem or treating a case. Always remember the caveat: "Well, it depends…"

Finally, to all the trainees and other colleagues around the world who will read and benefit from this workbook: welcome to our field, and enjoy every minute of your training years and your future practice!

Stephen P. Kraft, MD, FRCSC
The Hospital for Sick Children
Toronto, Canada
February 2014

ABBREVIATIONS

AET: alternating esotropia
BIO: bilateral inferior oblique
BIOAT: bilateral inferior oblique anterior transposition
BIR: bilateral inferior rectus
BLR: bilateral lateral rectus
BMR: bilateral medial rectus
BSR: bilateral superior rectus
ccET: esotropia with glasses
DEP: double elevator palsy
DRS: Duane retraction syndrome
ET: esotropia
EUA: examination under anesthesia
EX: exophoria
FD: forced ductions
HT: hypertropia
IO: inferior oblique
IR: inferior rectus
LET: left esotropia
LHT: left hypertropia
LIO: left inferior oblique
LIR: left inferior rectus
LLR: left lateral rectus
LMR: left medial rectus
LR: lateral rectus
LSO: left superior oblique
LSR: left superior rectus
LXT: left exotropia
MR: medial rectus
OA: overaction
OCT: ocular coherence tomography
OD: right eye
OS: left eye
OU: both eyes

PD: prism diopter
RET: right esotropia
RHT: right hypertropia
RhypoT: right hypotropia
RIO: right inferior oblique
RIOAT: right inferior oblique anterior transposition
RIR: right inferior rectus
RLR: right lateral rectus
RMR: right medial rectus
RSO: right superior oblique
RSR: right superior rectus
RXT: right exotropia
scET: esotropia without correction
SO: superior oblique
SR: superior rectus
VA: visual acuity
XT: exotropia
XT': exotropia at near

1

Approach to Strabismus Surgery Decision Making

Leonard B. Nelson, MD, MBA

Strabismus is one of the most common eye problems in pediatric ophthalmology. This misalignment may be manifest in all fields of gaze or only in certain fields; may be constant or intermittent; and may present at distance, near, or both. Early detection of strabismus in children is essential for the restoration of proper alignment of the visual axes, prevention of amblyopia, resolution of secondary anomalous head positions, and establishment of binocular vision. To proceed through the decision-making process in treating strabismus disorders, whether medically or surgically, it is imperative that a thorough history and examination be properly obtained. The history should include the patient's perceived strabismus condition, whether the deviation is constant or intermittent (and if intermittent, how frequent), associated symptoms such as diplopia, the presence of anomalous head position (old photographs may be useful for establishing onset), previous strabismus or amblyopia treatment, previous strabismus surgery (including operative reports if possible), and any concomitant systemic or ocular disorders. A complete ocular examination should be conducted, including dilated fundoscopy and cycloplegic refraction. Particular attention should be given to visual acuity testing, sensory testing, duction and version testing, and measurements of alignment in all relevant fields of gaze.

Nelson LB, Levin AV, eds.
The Wills Eye Strabismus Surgery Handbook (pp 1-5).
© 2015 Taylor & Francis Group.

One can also fit the treatment objectives into 1 or more of the following 4 categories: (1) improving prognosis, (2) improving function, (3) relieving symptoms, and (4) constructing a more normal appearance.[1] If the proposed treatment cannot be expected to improve any of these 4 categories, it should be questioned.

A decision to perform strabismus surgery to improve prognosis should be based on the knowledge of the course of the untreated disorder. For instance, reducing the duration of congenital esotropia before strabismus surgery improves long-term ocular motility and sensory outcomes.[2] In young children with a congenital fourth-nerve palsy and head tilt, reducing the duration of the disorder by strabismus surgery may eliminate the acquired facial asymmetry that has been observed in untreated patients.[3]

Another important reason to correct strabismus is to improve a patient's function. For instance, adults who have esotropia have a reduced field of binocular vision. After strabismus surgery, there is an expansion of the binocular visual field, which can have a significant impact on a patient's ability to drive and perform other daily activities.[4] Strabismus surgery that substantially reduces the deviation in congenital esotropia improves fine motor skills and visually directed reaching and grasping.[5]

The elimination or amelioration of annoying symptoms is a reasonable and justifiable rationale for strabismus surgery. Diplopia can be debilitating and have a profound effect on an individual's ability to perform activities of daily living. Correction of the strabismus that causes diplopia can allow patients to resume their normal activities. Abnormal or compensatory head positions may develop with a variety of strabismus conditions, including Duane syndrome, Brown syndrome, superior oblique palsy, and nystagmus. The long-term effects of an abnormal head position can result in changes in the musculoskeletal structures of the face or neck, psychosocial consequences, and/or difficulty in properly wearing glasses. Therefore, correction of a condition causing a significant abnormal head position is appropriately indicated.

Strabismus, itself, even without an abnormal head posture, can cause significant psychosocial problems for the affected individual.[6] These patients often report that the strabismus caused them embarrassment preoperatively and that they had trouble making eye contact; they therefore tended to develop mannerisms to camouflage their strabismus.[6] These problems arise partly because persons with strabismus may be perceived as having a lower level of intelligence. Strabismus surgery to restore ocular alignment is not merely cosmetic; it often has a significant effect on patients' self-esteem and self-confidence.[6] It is a reconstructive procedure to change an abnormal condition and appearance to be more normal.

After a complete and thorough history and ocular examination for a strabismus condition, a medical treatment plan should be prescribed if indicated. For example, a child with esotropia and hyperopia may be treated successfully with glasses to correct the hyperopia. Amblyopia is often best treated before proceeding to strabismus surgery and may occasionally result in improved alignment without surgery. If the initial examination shows that a medical treatment is not indicated or a medical treatment that was initiated is not successful, then a surgical approach can be offered if appropriate. It is preferable to discuss the surgical approach in the presence of the patient and, for children, the parents. The decision should not be a "stereotyped production" but adapted to the proposed surgical plan as well as to the personality of the patient and, in the case of a child, the views of the family.[7] The primary objectives in discussing the plan are to provide the proper information on the surgical procedure, including the anticipated final outcome, and to dispel any misconceptions about the surgical approach.[7] For instance, in a patient with esotropia who has both an accommodative and a nonaccomodative component, the strabismus surgeon's explanation should clearly indicate that the purpose of the surgery is to eliminate the nonaccomodative component. Following the surgery, eyeglasses will still be required to compensate for the accommodative component. The primary surgical result for a sixth-nerve palsy is to eliminate the primary-position esotropia and diplopia. However, it is important for the patient to understand that the abduction deficiency, esotropia, and diplopia in gaze toward the ipsilateral lateral rectus will most likely remain. Some strabismus disorders are particularly confusing to the patient and/or the parents in terms of which eye actually has the condition requiring surgery. For example, parents of patients with Duane retraction syndrome type 1 of the left eye very often believe that the right eye has esotropia. This occurs because when the patient looks to the left, the right eye adducts normally while the left eye has reduced abduction. In that position, it appears to the parents that the right eye is esotropic and therefore requires surgery. It is important to resolve this confusion regarding the clinical picture and to explain why the apparently "normal eye" is the one requiring surgery.

Another aspect of the discussion is to provide the individual or family with a realistic and thorough prognosis and expected outcome of the proposed surgery. Therefore, the strabismus surgeon must explain carefully and fully the risks, benefits, limitations, and alternatives to surgery. The most common "risk" of strabismus surgery is failure to achieve long-standing alignment or completely ameliorate the associated symptoms, such as diplopia or an anomalous head position. More complex strabismus conditions—such as previous strabismus surgery, subnormal vision, cerebral palsy, craniofacial syndromes, extraocular muscle trauma, or large delays between the onset and intervention for the condition—make the outcome less predictable. It is important that the patient and/or family understand that strabismus exists within a complex visual system and that the mere moving of extraocular muscles cannot always totally resolve the condition or its associated symptoms. The benefits of strabismus surgery include reducing or eliminating the deviation and/or the associated symptoms. Once it is determined that strabismus surgery is indicated, few alternatives exist. These may include, in specific circumstances, monocular occlusion, fogging, patching prisms, or botulinum toxin injections. The surgeon should also describe in an understandable manner how the strabismus surgery is performed. The use of a model of the eye or other visual aids is helpful in this regard.

The decision-making process in developing a surgical approach to many strabismus disorders is often relatively straightforward, although some cases may be more complex.[8] For instance, if a 6-month-old child has a large alternating and constant esotropia, the decision to perform a large bimedial recession would be seconded by most pediatric ophthalmologists. However, if a patient has had multiple previous strabismus surgeries, the decision about how to proceed surgically becomes more involved. In planning strabismus surgery, it is necessary to determine whether to operate on one or both eyes, whether to perform a unilateral recession or resection, whether to do a recession and resection on an antagonistic muscle, whether to perform bilateral symmetrical surgery, and the amount of recession or resection to perform for a specific degree of deviation. These decisions are based on the size of the preoperative deviation, the presence of amblyopia, a history of previous strabismus surgery, and the surgeon's own guidelines.

Although the surgical approach to each strabismus condition may vary, there are certain specific guidelines to which most pediatric ophthalmologists would agree. Amblyopia or poor vision in one eye is an important factor when strabismus surgery is being planned. There is a very small (less than 1%, but still definite) risk of vision loss as a result of strabismus surgery; however, most pediatric ophthalmologists operate on the eye with more limited vision.[8] When the vision in both eyes is nearly equal, there are situations in which the surgeon would prefer to operate on the dominant eye yet be overruled by the patient for fear of a possible complication to the perceived "normal" eye.[9] For example, if a patient already had a recess-resect procedure on one eye, operating on the previously untouched muscles of the other eye might be a preferable strategy. If a patient with strabismus has normal rotation in an eye that has an encircling band from a previous retinal detachment procedure, strabismus surgery would be easier if surgery were performed on the opposite eye. In general, recessions are usually preferred to resections. A recession procedure is easier and therefore faster to perform than a resection. Recession is also less damaging to the muscle. Bleeding may be more common in a resection because of the need to excise muscle within its belly as opposed to the tendinous portion, which is removed in a recession procedure. Finally, recessions tend to have a more acceptable cosmetic appearance postoperatively than resections, in which a salmon-pink, fleshy, thickened appearance of the subconjunctival tissue occasionally remains apparent.

Learning how to manage strabismus, both medically and surgically, begins during residency and continues through fellowship training and beyond. Surgeons should continually review their outcomes to adjust their surgical dosing and operation selection accordingly. The decision-making process in strabismus surgery requires years of experience. When he or she is called upon to obtain the necessary measurements from a difficult and uncooperative child, an experienced examiner's skills can be invaluable and essential for optimizing outcomes. Complex strabismus conditions require not only the formulation of an appropriate surgical plan but also a surgeon who is prepared to modify and adjust his or her initial plans in the operating room, if necessary, on the basis of the given anatomy, forced ductions, and other factors. Finally, the surgeon must be able to properly communicate the anticipated surgical outcome in a skillful and compassionate manner.

REFERENCES

1. Calhoun JH, Nelson LB, Harley RD. *Atlas of Pediatric Ophthalmic Surgery.* Philadelphia, PA: WB Saunders; 1987.
2. Birch EE, Stager DR Sr. Long-term motor and sensory outcomes after early surgery for infantile esotropia. *J AAPOS.* 2006;10(5):409-413.
3. Nelson LB, Olitsky SE. *Harley's Pediatric Ophthalmology.* 6th ed. Philadelphia, PA: Lippincott Williams & Wilkins; 2014.
4. Wortham E V, Greenwald MJ. Expanded binocular peripheral visual fields following surgery for esotropia. *J Pediatr Ophthalmol Strabismus.* 1989;26(3):109-112.
5. Rogers GL, Chazan S, Fellows R, Tsou BH. Strabismus surgery and its effect upon infant development in congenital esotropia. *Ophthalmology.* 1982;89(5):479-483.
6. Nelson BA, Gunton KB, Lasker JN, Nelson LB, Drohan LA. The psychosocial aspects of strabismus in teenagers and adults and the impact of surgical correction. *J AAPOS.* 2008;12(1):72-76.e1.
7. Parks MM. *Atlas of Strabismus Surgery.* Philadelphia, PA: Harper and Row; 1983.
8. Wagner RS, Nelson LB. Complications following strabismus surgery. In: Nelson LB, Wagner RS, eds. *Strabismus Surgery International Ophthalmology Clinics.* Boston, MA: Little, Brown, and Co; 1985:171-178.
9. Coats DK, Olitsky SE. *Strabismus Surgery and Its Complications.* New York, NY: Springer; 2007.

2

Esotropia

Scott Olitsky, MD

Correction of esotropia is one of the most common surgical procedures performed by pediatric ophthalmologists. Before surgery, the patient should be given a prescription for the full cycloplegic refraction to correct any significant hyperopia that may be contributing to the deviation. In addition, most pediatric ophthalmologists will stress the need to correct any amblyopia that is present prior to recommending surgery. Surgery may be indicated when the deviation continues to be too large to allow for the development of some level of binocular vision; this will help in maintaining future ocular alignment. It may mean that surgery is indicated when the deviation is larger than 8 prism diopters. Other ophthalmologists believe that surgery should be performed only if the esodeviation is cosmetically significant, as determined by the patient, family, or both. These physicians feel that there is no functional deficit that can be demonstrated consistently in a real-world situation in patients who do not have peripheral fusion, as would be present with monofixation syndrome.

When surgery is indicated, most strabismus surgeons prefer to perform a medial rectus recession when possible. Recession tends to require less time and leads to less postoperative discomfort in most patients. Bilateral recessions are performed for larger deviations, and unilateral recessions may be performed for smaller amounts of crossing. For cases in which surgery was previously performed on the medial rectus muscles, a lateral rectus resection is usually chosen. In cases of unilaterally decreased vision,

Nelson LB, Levin AV, eds.
The Wills Eye Strabismus Surgery Handbook (pp 7-14).
© 2015 Taylor & Francis Group.

a lateral rectus resection may be combined with a medial rectus recession of the affected eye.

Some patients with esotropia also have other concurrent strabismus-related disorders, which may include oblique muscle dysfunction, A and V patterns, dissociated vertical deviation, and high accommodative convergence/accommodation ratio esotropia, which can be treated at the same time that the esotropia is being corrected. The following cases demonstrate some of the most common scenarios that the surgeon may face in treating patients with esotropia.

Case 1

Congenital esotropia. ET = 70 at distance and near fixation.

Surgeon 1: Recess the BMR 7 mm.
Surgeon 2: Recess the BMR 6.5 mm.
Surgeon 3: Recess the BMR 7 mm.

Case 2

Congenital esotropia. ET = 40 at distance and near fixation.

Surgeon 1: Recess the BMR 5.5 mm.
Surgeon 2: Recess the BMR 5.5 mm.
Surgeon 3: Recess the BMR 5.5 mm.

Case 3

Congenital esotropia. ET = 50 at distance and near fixation. OA BIO, no pattern.

Surgeon 1: Recess the BMR 6 mm; would perform bilateral IO myectomy if overaction greater than +2 or cosmetically apparent.
Surgeon 2: Recess the BMR 5.5 mm; recess the IO OU 14 mm without myectomy.
Surgeon 3: Recess the BMR 6 mm; recess the BIO between 10 and 14 mm depending on degree of IO overaction, at least +2.

Case 4

ET = 30 at distance and near fixation. Upgaze = 20, downgaze = 35. BIO, normal.

Surgeon 1: Recess the BMR 4.5 mm.

Surgeon 2: Recess the BMR 4.5 mm with a half-tendon-width inferior displacement of both.

Surgeon 3: Recess the BMR 4.5 mm with a half-tendon-width inferior displacement of both.

Case 5

ET = 25 at distance and near fixation. Upgaze = 10, downgaze = 35. OA BIO.

Surgeon 1: Recess the BMR 4 mm; BIO myectomy.
Surgeon 2: Recess the BMR 4 mm; recess BIO 14 mm without myectomy.
Surgeon 3: Recess the BMR 4 mm; recess BIO 14 mm without myectomy.

Case 6

ET = 25 at distance and near fixation. Upgaze = 10, downgaze = 35. BIO, normal.

Surgeon 1: Recess the BMR 4 mm with a half-tendon-width inferior displacement.

Surgeon 2: Recess the BMR 4 mm with 1-tendon-width inferior displacement.

Surgeon 3: Recess the BMR 4 mm with 1-tendon-width inferior displacement.

Case 7

ET = 20 at distance and near fixation. Refractory amblyopia OD.

Surgeon 1: Recess the RMR 5.5 mm.
Surgeon 2: Recess the RMR 5.5 mm.
Surgeon 3: Recess the RMR 3.5 mm; resect or plicate the RLR 4 mm.

Case 8

ET = 30 at distance and near fixation. Refractory amblyopia OD.

Surgeon 1: Recess the RMR 4.5 mm; resect the RLR 5.5 mm.
Surgeon 2: Recess the RMR 7 mm.
Surgeon 3: Recess the RMR 4.5 mm; resect or plicate the RLR 5.5 mm.

Case 9

ET = 50 at distance and near fixation. Refractory amblyopia OD.

Surgeon 1: Recess the RMR 6 mm; resect the RLR 7 mm.
Surgeon 2: Recess the RMR 6.5 mm; resect the RLR 8 mm.
Surgeon 3: Recess the RMR 6 mm; resect or plicate the RLR 6 mm.

Case 10

EX = 0 at distance fixation, ET = 25 at near fixation in a 5-year-old child. Refraction plano.

Surgeon 1: I would not operate on this child but would give bifocals: plano with a +3 add. Would specify flat-top bifocal with the segment line to bisect the pupil.
Surgeon 2: Recess the BMR 4 mm.
Surgeon 3: I would not operate on this patient but would continue bifocals: plano with a +3 bifocal addition.

Case 11

ET = 20 at distance fixation, ET = 35 at near. fixation Refraction plano.

Surgeon 1: Recess the BMR 4 mm.
Surgeon 2: Recess the BMR 5 mm.
Surgeon 3: Recess the BMR 5 mm.

Case 12

ET = 30 at distance fixation, ET = 55 at near fixation. Refraction plano.

Surgeon 1: Recess the BMR 4.5 mm.
Surgeon 2: Recess the BMR 6 mm.
Surgeon 3: Recess the BMR 6 mm.

Case 13

ccET = 20 at distance and near. Wearing +2 OU.

Surgeon 1: Recess the RMR 5.5 mm.
Surgeon 2: Recess the BMR 3.5 mm.
Surgeon 3: Recess the BMR 3 mm.

Case 14

ccET = 20 at distance and near. fixation Wearing +9 OU.

Surgeon 1: Recess the MR unilaterally 6 mm.
Surgeon 2: Recess the BMR 4 mm OU.
Surgeon 3: Recess the BMR 3.5 mm.

Case 15

A 10-year-old child with ccET = 0 at distance fixation, cc bifocal ET = 0 at near fixation, cc without bifocal ET = 20, scET = 25 at distance, scET = 45 at near. Wants to stop using bifocal.

Surgeon 1: I would not perform surgery in this patient. I would attempt to slowly taper the bifocal correction to determine if the patient could maintain alignment. If unable to taper the bifocal correction and the child has been successfully wearing bifocal, I would try switching to a progressive bifocal.
Surgeon 2: Recess the MR 3.5 mm OU.
Surgeon 3: I would not operate but would continue bifocal glasses.

Case 16

ccET = 0 at distance fixation, cc bifocal ET = 20 at near fixation, cc without bifocal ET = 40. Bifocal = +3.50 OU.

Surgeon 1: I would not perform surgery in this patient.
Surgeon 2: Recess the BMR 5.5 mm.
Surgeon 3: Recess the BMR 3 mm or Faden procedure BMR.

Case 17

High accommodative convergence/accommodation ratio ET initially controlled with bifocal glasses but now ccET = 20 at distance fixation, cc bifocal ET = 30 at near fixation.

Surgeon 1: Recess the RMR 5.5 mm.
Surgeon 2: Recess the BMR 4.5 mm.
Surgeon 3: Recess the BMR 4.5 mm.

DISCUSSION

These cases provide examples of how experienced surgeons might treat a variety of scenarios that are commonly seen in patients requiring surgery for esotropia. The surgeons generally agreed that they would perform bilateral, symmetric, medial rectus recession for cases in which the patient had not had previous surgery and there was not a significant difference in vision between the eyes. Standard tables are available in most strabismus textbooks that provide guidelines for the amount of surgery to perform. Many surgeons will examine their results using these guidelines and may adjust the amount of surgery they perform accordingly. For large angles of esotropia, as in Case 1, some surgeons will perform 3-muscle surgery in which they do smaller recessions on the medial rectus muscles and add a resection of a lateral rectus muscle. In the past, it was thought that larger recessions could lead to a duction deficit, but this has not been shown to be true. Surgeons who perform 3-muscle surgery on patients with large-angle esotropia will often do so because they feel their results are better than when they perform 2-muscle surgery.

Many patients with congenital, or infantile, esotropia will demonstrate overaction of the inferior oblique, as is seen in Case 3. To treat the inferior oblique overaction, all 3 surgeons would perform a weakening procedure on the inferior oblique at the time of surgery to correct the esotropia. There are a number of ways to weaken the inferior oblique, including recession, myotomy, and myectomy. The inferior oblique is commonly recessed either 10 or 14 mm depending on the amount of overaction present. Each of these procedures can effectively treat overaction. Some surgeons prefer one procedure over another depending on the amount of overaction they are treating. ATIO may provide correction of larger amounts of overaction. It can also be used to treat DVD, which occurs in many patients with congenital esotropia as well. Therefore, it is a procedure that is often used whenever inferior oblique overaction and DVD are both present. In addition, there is some evidence that ATIO may help to prevent the development of DVD, leading some surgeons to perform ATIO in any patient with a history of congenital esotropia when inferior oblique overaction is being treated regardless of the magnitude of the existing overaction.

A V-pattern esotropia exists when the deviation is larger in downgaze and smaller in upgaze. A V pattern often occurs in patients with esotropia secondary to overaction of the inferior oblique muscles. In these cases, surgery on the inferior oblique muscles will generally be effective in collapsing the pattern (eg, Case 5). However, V patterns also occur with normal oblique function. Surgery on the inferior obliques in this situation could convert the

V pattern into an A pattern. Therefore, displacement of the rectus muscles is used in these cases (eg, Case 4). The muscle is generally displaced a half tendon width. Some surgeons may displace the muscle a full tendon width for larger patterns (eg, Case 6).

When one eye sees poorly due to amblyopia or an organic abnormality, surgery is generally restricted to the poorly seeing eye. For larger deviations, surgery would typically involve a recess/resect procedure in the amblyopic eye (eg, Case 9). For small-to-moderate deviations, a larger recession of the medial rectus without a simultaneous lateral rectus resection is used by some surgeons (eg, Cases 7 and 8). This may be an attractive option because it spares a lateral rectus muscle if future surgery is needed. An individual surgeon will generally have an upper limit of esotropia for which he or she will perform a single medial rectus recession before adding a resection to the procedure. The concern is that performing a recession that is too large may lead to an adduction deficit. Some surgeons will accept a small postoperative deficit in order to limit surgery to just one muscle.

Some patients with esotropia will demonstrate a larger deviation at near fixation than is present at distance. Several options exist for the treatment of excess esotropia at near fixation. Most pediatric ophthalmologists will use bifocal lenses to treat the excess esotropia if the distance deviation is small enough to allow for the development of fusion. Others believe that surgery is a better option for these patients. In Case 10, two of the surgeons would opt for bifocals, given that the patient has good alignment at distance fixation. When the distance deviation is too large to allow for the development of fusion, surgery is indicated to align the eyes at both distance and near fixation (eg, Cases 11, 12, and 17). Some surgeons will target the amount of surgery for the distance fixation and then place the patient into a bifocal for any residual near esotropia, as Surgeon 1 would do in these cases. Other surgeons will operate for the full deviation that is present at near fixation because a number of studies have shown that these patients can to do well without the risk of consecutive exotropia. A posterior fixation suture (or Faden operation) may be used by some surgeons for this purpose. A third option may include operating for a deviation somewhere between the distance and near deviation to increase the chance of alignment at near fixation if there is a concern about producing a consecutive exotropia. If a residual esotropia remains, it can then be treated with bifocals. If the patient is already in bifocals, surgery may be suggested to allow for alignment without the need for bifocals or even eyeglasses if the level of hyperopia is small. Cases 15 and 16 are examples of when surgery can be performed for this purpose.

When a significant distance esotropia remains after a patient has been placed in his or her full hyperopic correction, as determined by a cycloplegic refraction, surgery may be required. This type of esotropia is termed a *mixed-mechanism esotropia*, and the residual esotropia that occurs is the nonaccommodative component. As seen in Cases 13 and 14, surgery may be offered to correct the nonaccommodative portion of the crossing. In Case 13, all 3 surgeons would operate only for the amount of crossing that is present with the eyeglasses in place. This patient has a low degree of hyperopia, and, depending on the amount of esotropia that occurs without the glasses, it may be possible to perform surgery that will allow good alignment with no need for corrective lenses. Because of the risk of undercorrection in patients with mixed-mechanism esotropia, surgeons may operate for a larger deviation than exists with glasses and then reduce the amount of hyperopic correction if an overcorrection occurs. This is seen in Case 14. Surgeons 1 and 2 would do a larger amount of surgery than may be needed for the nonaccommodative esotropia with the thought that adjusting the prescription could not be done to deal with an undercorrection but that it could be done to reduce an overcorrection.

These cases show commonly encountered examples of esotropia requiring surgical correction. They also demonstrate that a number of good solutions exist for treating these patients.

Suggested Readings

Arnoldi K. Long-term surgical outcome of partially accommodative esotropia. *Am Orthop J.* 2002;52(1):75-84.

Dickmann A, Petroni S, Salerni A, et al. Effect of vertical transposition of the medial rectus muscle on primary position alignment in infantile esotropia with A- or V-pattern strabismus. *J AAPOS.* 2011;15(1):14-16.

Kushner BJ. Fifteen-year outcome of surgery for the near angle in patients with accommodative esotropia and a high accommodative convergence to accommodation ratio. *Arch Ophthalmol.* 2001;119(8):1150-1153.

Rajavi Z, Ferdosi A, Eslamdoust M, et al. The prevalence of reoperation and related risk factors among patients with congenital esotropia. *J Pediatr Ophthalmol Strabismus.* 2013;50:53-59.

Vroman DT, Hutchinson AK, Saunders RA, Wilson ME. Two-muscle surgery for congenital esotropia: rate of reoperation in patients with small versus large angles of deviation. *J AAPOS.* 2000;4(5):267-270.

3

Exotropia

Daniel T. Weaver, MD

Exodeviations are less common than esodeviations by a ratio of 1:3 in the United States and overall account for approximately 25% of the cases of strabismus in young children. These statistics vary in different parts of the world, with exodeviations appearing at higher frequencies in Asia and in locations proximate to the equator. Exotropia generally appears in the first few years of life and is slightly more common in girls. Some 60% to 70% of normal newborn infants have a transient exodeviation that resolves by 4 to 6 months of age.

Exotropia can be categorized as divergence excess (greater deviation at distance than at near fixation), convergence insufficiency (greater deviation at near than at distance fixation), or basic exotropia (deviation same at distance and at near fixation). In some patients with exotropia who have strong functional convergence and variability in the angle of deviation measured on the prolonged alternate cover test, a patch test may be indicated. The patch test consists of placing an occlusive patch over one eye for approximately 30 minutes and then measuring the deviation without permitting the patient to begin binocular fusion. The patch test eliminates functional convergence, allowing the full deviation to be measured. The exodeviations can also be categorized as exophoria, intermittent exotropia, or constant exotropia. Exophoria is a tendency for the visual axes to diverge, which is held in check by fusion. Exotropia can present initially as an intermittent deviation and can later progress to a more constant deviation. Children with intermittent exotropia

Nelson LB, Levin AV, eds.
The Wills Eye Strabismus Surgery Handbook (pp 15-24).
© 2015 Taylor & Francis Group.

will often close one eye in bright sunlight. There have been many proposed mechanisms to explain monocular eye closure in sunlight; it may be to avoid diplopia or reduce photophobia. A history of intermittent exotropia provided by the patient's parents should usually be considered valid because the office examination may not reveal a manifest deviation when the child is alert and well rested. Intermittent exodeviations tend to become more apparent when the child is tired or unwell. Assessing control and degree of intermittent exotropia may require repeated office visits. Asthenopic symptoms and headache are all commonly noted in the exotropic child. A short attention span in school has been noted in some children, but this perception may be more due to the deviation being noted by the teachers. Eye drifting for more than 50% of waking hours and manifest deviation noted without cover testing mandate consideration of surgery.

Office evaluation should include measurements at distance and near fixation, and in the nine cardinal positions of gaze with refractive correction in place. Stereopsis should be assessed. It is important to document ARC in adults with long-standing exotropia because many of these patients will experience postoperative diplopia and must be warned of this possibility. With ARC, the exotropic eye develops a second foveation (fixation) point temporal to the anatomic fovea; following surgical realignment, this eye is perceived by the brain to be in an esotropic position. Fortunately, diplopia in this situation is usually temporary. It is important to recognize lateral incomitance, usually a lesser exodeviation in side gaze, to prevent a postoperative overcorrection in lateral gaze. A and V patterns commonly occur in exotropia because of oblique muscle overaction or underaction. Vertical offsets of the medial and lateral recti can be utilized to address this situation during horizontal muscle-weakening procedures. Prism adaptation—the progressive use of Fresnel prisms with sequential measurements at serial visits to ensure that the maximum deviation is exposed—is used by some pediatric ophthalmologists in the preoperative management of exotropia.

Case 1

Infantile extropia. XT at distance and near fixation = 70 PD.

Surgeon 1: Recess the BLR 9 mm.

Surgeon 2: Recess the BLR 10 mm if younger than 12 months. If older, recess the BLR 9.0 mm and resect 1 MR 6.0 mm in the eye that appears to be deviated more frequently.

Surgeon 3: Recess the BLR 11 mm.

Case 2

Infantile exotropia. XT at distance and near fixation = 40 PD.

Surgeon 1: Recess the BLR 7 mm.
Surgeon 2: Recess the BLR 8 mm.
Surgeon 3: Recess the BLR 8.5 mm.

Case 3

LXT at distance and near fixation = 18 PD.

Surgeon 1: Recess the LLR 7.5 mm.
Surgeon 2: Recess the LLR 7.5 mm.
Surgeon 3: Recess the LLR 7.5 mm.

Case 4

XT at distance and near fixation = 30 PD. Upgaze 35, downgaze 25. IOs, normal.

Surgeon 1: Recess the BLR 7 mm.
Surgeon 2: Recess the BLR 7 mm.
Surgeon 3: Recess the BLR 7 mm with a half-tendon-width superior displacement.

Case 5

XT at distance and near fixation = 25 PD. Upgaze 35, downgaze 20.

Surgeon 1: Recess the BLR 6 mm with BIO distal 5-mm myectomy at the IO insertion.
Surgeon 2: Recess the BLR 6 mm. If there is IO overaction greater than or equal to +3, recess the BIO (without myectomy) to the Crawford position (6 mm posterior to the lateral border of the inferior rectus muscle insertion). If less IO OA, operate only on the lateral recti. In addition, a young patient will grow taller, and a small V pattern will become less noticeable. Therefore, if the child is 5 years of age or older, I would not operate on the IOs.
Surgeon 3: Recess the BLR 6 mm and recess the BIO to the Crawford position (6 mm posterior to the lateral border of the insertion of the inferior rectus muscle).

Case 6

XT at distance and near fixation = 25 PD. Upgaze 45, downgaze 10. BIO OA.

Surgeon 1: Recess the BLR 6 mm and BIO 5-mm myectomy at the insertion.

Surgeon 2: Recess the BLR 6 mm and recess the BIO to the Crawford position (6 mm posterior to the lateral border of the insertion of the inferior rectus muscle).

Surgeon 3: Recess the BLR 6 mm OU and recess the BIO to the Crawford position (6 mm posterior to the lateral border of the insertion of the inferior rectus muscle).

Case 7

RXT at distance and near fixation = 20 PD. Refractory amblyopia OD.

Surgeon 1: Recess the RLR 8 mm.

Surgeon 2: Recess the RLR 8 mm.

Surgeon 3: Recess the RLR 5 mm and resect the RMR 4 mm.

Case 8

RXT at distance and near fixation = 30 PD. Refractory amblyopia OD.

Surgeon 1: Recess the RLR 6.5 mm and resect the RMR 5 mm.

Surgeon 2: Recess the RLR 7 mm and resect the RMR 6 mm. Another option would be to recess the RLR 10 mm to leave the MR untouched in the event that further surgery is needed in the future.

Surgeon 3: Recess the RLR 7 mm and resect the RMR 6 mm.

Case 9

RXT at distance and near fixation = 50 PD. Refractory amblyopia OD.

Surgeon 1: Recess the RLR 8.5 mm and resect the RMR 6.5 mm.

Surgeon 2: Recess the RLR 9 mm and resect the RMR 7 mm.

Surgeon 3: Recess the RLR 9 mm and resect the RMR 7 mm.

Case 10

XT at distance fixation = 30 PD, at near fixation = 45, plano refraction.

Surgeon 1: Recess the BLR 7.5 mm.

Surgeon 2: Recess 1 LR 7 mm and resect the ipsilateral MR 6 mm in the eye that appears to be deviating most frequently.

Surgeon 3: Resect the BMR 5.5 mm.

Case 11

XT at distance fixation = 45 PD, at near fixation = 15, plano refraction.

Surgeon 1: I would perform a 30-minute patch test in the office on the eye that appears to be deviating most frequently. If the distance/near disparity remains, I would recess the BLR 7 mm. If after the patch test the near deviation increases, recess the BLR 7.5 mm.

Surgeon 2: Recess the BLR 8 mm.

Surgeon 3: Recess the BLR 9 mm.

Case 12

No XT at distance fixation, XT at near fixation = 20 PD. Failed orthoptics and prisms.

Surgeon 1: Resect the BMR 4 mm.

Surgeon 2: Would not recommend surgery because of risk of diplopia at distance. Try fogging 1 bifocal lens.

Surgeon 3: Would not recommend surgery because of risk of diplopia at distance. If no suppression by Worth 4-dot testing, could use Bangerter foil on 1 lens for reading.

Case 13

XT at distance fixation = 10 PD, at near fixation = 30 PD.

Surgeon 1: Recess the BLR 5 mm.

Surgeon 2: First try orthoptic exercises for convergence insufficiency and prism in eyeglasses if diplopia is present at distance because of the small deviation. If this fails, resect a single MR 4 mm in the eye that appears deviated most frequently.

Surgeon 3: If divergence amplitudes are normal, resect BMR 3 mm. If divergence amplitudes are abnormal, resect a single MR 5 mm in the eye that appears deviated most frequently.

Case 14

XT at distance and near fixation = 35 PD, in side gaze to each side = 25 PD.

Surgeon 1: Recess the BLR 5 mm.

Surgeon 2: Recess the BLR 7 mm.

Surgeon 3: Recess the BLR 6 mm.

Case 15

XT at distance and near fixation = 30 PD. Wearing –9.50 sphere eyeglasses.

Surgeon 1: Recess the BLR 7 mm.

Surgeon 2: Recess a single LR 8.5 mm in the eye that appears deviated most frequently.

Surgeon 3: Recess the BLR 6 mm.

DISCUSSION

Large-angle infantile exotropia, as in Cases 1 and 2, is now treated with early surgery by most pediatric ophthalmologists. An existing disparity in fixation preference is addressed with preoperative patching, but early fusion is the goal in managing these patients, as in the outcome desired for infantile large-angle esotropia. Large lateral rectus muscle recessions are employed. Some strabismus surgeons prefer not to add a third muscle initially because of the risk of overcorrection and instead delay it for a second procedure after waiting 3 to 4 months, intervening with the third muscle only if residual exotropia persists. Early overcorrection (esotropia) is frequently noted and many times will correct itself without patching or further intervention. Significant overcorrection (> 15 PD), persisting longer than 6 to 8 weeks, may require patching or subsequent surgery. In my experience, BLR muscle recessions of less than 10 mm with a deviation of 70 PD in infantile exotropia will result in undercorrection and require further surgery. I would select a 10-mm BLR muscle recession in Case 1 and a 9-mm BLR muscle recession in Case 2. Variations in the surgical dose suggested by the 3 surgeons may reflect differences in surgical technique.

Unilateral small-angle (< 25 PD) exotropia is often amenable to unilateral lateral rectus muscle recession. Standard doses for exotropia may result in early undercorrection. I now utilize larger doses (eg, 9 mm for 20 PD) and prefer BLR muscle weakening for deviations larger than this. The approach to V-pattern exotropia depends on several factors, including the size of the pattern and inferior oblique action. The V pattern in Case 4 is not large, and inferior oblique function is normal. Recession of each lateral rectus muscle of 7 mm is a reasonable approach, but adding a half-tendon-width supraplacement of the lateral rectus tendons could also work well. I would favor the latter approach, as suggested by Surgeon 3, to optimize alignment in primary position and downgaze. In Case 5, the V pattern is again mild, but I would still advocate bilateral inferior oblique weakening to the Crawford position (6 mm posterior to the lateral border of the insertion of the inferior rectus muscle) combined with a 6-mm bilateral lateral rectus recession, as advocated by Surgeons 1 and 3. There have been numerous approaches to surgical weakening of the inferior oblique muscle; these techniques vary in terms of muscle positioning in regard to the desired potency of the recession. Others have also described the different indications for inferior oblique recession vs myectomy. One distinct advantage of the recession technique is that the muscle can be located at future reoperation if there is a need for further revision of the inferior oblique.

V-pattern exotropia often results from oblique muscle dysfunction. Inferior oblique overaction with or without coexisting superior oblique underaction can result in significant differences in the exodeviation in up- and downgaze to create a V pattern. Symmetrical inferior oblique weakening to the Crawford position (6 mm posterior to the lateral border of the insertion of the inferior rectus muscle) is commonly combined with lateral rectus muscle recession and does not require adjustment of the usual dose for lateral rectus muscle recession employed in primary position. Case 6 demonstrates a very significant V-pattern exotropia and may even represent a bilateral congenital superior oblique paresis. Whether the superior oblique muscles are underacting in this case is not mentioned, but this should be investigated with extraocular muscle versions and fundus excyclotorsion assessment in the clinic and superior oblique tendon forced duction testing intraoperatively. This patient might require superior oblique strengthening as a primary or secondary procedure, but here we are not given enough information to make that determination. However, the surgical approaches outlined by the 3 surgeons are very safe and reasonable first steps.

Approximately 50% of children with poor vision in one eye and strabismus will become esotropic, and the other half will become exotropic. Surgery on the amblyopic eye is always a safer choice because the good eye is not put at risk. Parents usually find this preferable as well. Unilateral lateral rectus muscle recession for smaller deviations (25 PD or less) and recess-resect procedures for larger deviations are common approaches. As reoperation in exotropic patients is common (usually for recurrent exotropia), I prefer to touch only one muscle whenever possible in the event that reoperation should be needed. A small undercorrection following a unilateral 8-mm lateral rectus muscle recession for exotropia of 20 PD would be preferable to overcorrection in the setting of amblyopia; this is what I would perform in Case 7, as also proposed by Surgeons 1 and 2.

In patients with refractory amblyopia, overcorrection will often persist and is to be avoided if possible. For this reason, larger unilateral lateral rectus muscle recession may be considered for the treatment of deviations up to 30 PD. In Case 8, the dosage recommended by Surgeon 1 might result in undercorrection, but in this setting, that would not be a bad result. As suggested by Surgeon 2, a large unilateral lateral rectus muscle recession in this case might be the best option. In Case 9, Surgeons 2 and 3 are following logic similar to that in Case 8, utilizing standard dosage tables. Surgeon 1 has recommended a slightly reduced dose to prevent an overcorrection, which in such a case can result in intractable diplopia and a very unhappy patient. Preoperative red lens testing to identify ARC can potentially help to avoid this situation and make a small undercorrection more desirable. In this case, I would also favor a slight undercorrection and utilize the plan of Surgeon 1, but the plans of Surgeons 2 and 3 are also perfectly acceptable.

Convergence insufficiency exotropia with deviation greater at near fixation will sometimes respond to orthoptic vision therapy. This can be a very challenging clinical scenario. Paste-on or ground-in base in prism spectacles for use at near fixation works well for some patients. If surgery is required, bilateral lateral rectus muscle weakening for the distance deviation will generally lead to an undercorrection at near fixation. Kraft et al[1] have suggested a "biased" recess-resect with at least 1 mm more of medial rectus resection than lateral rectus recession. This may work well with an adjustable suture on the lateral rectus muscle to avoid undercorrection at near. In Case 10, I would favor resection of one medial rectus 6 mm with ipsilateral recession of the lateral rectus 6 mm, with the lateral rectus on an adjustable suture. Adjustable sutures can be useful in the surgical management of selected cases of exotropia. They give the surgeon a second chance for obtaining optimal alignment and are often helpful in preventing postoperative diplopia. Patient selection is critical, since some degree of postoperative cooperation is needed under topical anesthesia in the office. Some investigators have used adjustable sutures in children, but this requires returning to the operating room for further general anesthesia and is not routinely done by most pediatric ophthalmologists.

Divergence excess exotropia with deviation greater at distance fixation, as seen in Case 11, generally responds well to bilateral lateral rectus recession for the distance deviation. Overcorrection at near fixation does not usually occur in this setting.

Case 12 is a very difficult scenario. If the deviation at distance is orthophoric and orthoptic treatment has failed to improve symptoms, small medial rectus muscle resections for the deviation at near fixation may suffice. Lateral rectus muscle weakening in this setting commonly leads to overcorrection; if this is considered, adjustable sutures may be advisable. I would avoid operating on this patient, as also suggested by all 3 surgeons. In my experience, fogging one bifocal has worked, as also suggested by Surgeons 2 and 3 in this case. Case 13 is similar. Orthoptic exercises and/ or a prism trial would be my first option, as suggested by Surgeon 2. Lateral rectus muscle recession can result in diplopia at distance and would not be my first choice. Small medial rectus resections might provide the most predictable result. In this case, provided that nonsurgical options had failed, unilateral or bilateral medial rectus strengthening can be considered. Using an adjustable suture on one of the medial rectus muscles would provide an opportunity to examine the patient postoperatively to determine how much esodeviation at distance he or she can tolerate. Another alternative is a medial rectus muscle plication, which can also be placed on an adjustable suture. This procedure is easily reversible and can be adjusted. My choice would be a 4-mm resection of the right medial rectus muscle and a 4-mm plication of the left medial rectus muscle on an adjustable suture.

The presence of lateral incomitance must always be investigated in the setting of alternating exotropia. Some investigators have suggested an increased risk of overcorrection in these patients. For this reason, reducing the amount of recession by 0.5 mm per muscle may be advisable if the deviation in lateral gaze is significantly less than the deviation in primary position. I am less concerned about overcorrection in side gaze than I am with undercorrection in primary position. I would proceed with the plan of Surgeon 2 in this case.

The patient with exotropia and high refractive error poses a unique challenge that requires familiarity with Prentice's rule. Because of the prismatic effect of a highly myopic (or hyperopic) lens, adjustments must be made in the usual dosage of lateral rectus muscle recession in primary position. For a highly myopic lens, the base-out effect of the spectacle lens on the path of light into a laterally deviated eye leads to a reduction in the usual amount of recession needed because the measured exotropia through the eyeglasses is actually greater than the true deviation. For example, an exotropia of 30 PD (distance and near fixation) in a patient wearing −9.50 spectacles would require recession of the lateral rectus muscle for approximately 25 PD.

Postoperative management in exotropia requires close observation of ocular alignment, which is often esotropic in the first several weeks. Esodeviations up to 20 PD may resolve without intervention; some overcorrection is desirable by most experienced strabismus surgeons. Postoperative diplopia is common in children and adults and generally resolves. Esotropia of greater than 15 PD that persists for more than 6 to 8 weeks will often require reoperation; in young children, it can result in amblyopia and loss of bifoveal fixation and stereopsis. Overcorrection in adult patients may result in intractable diplopia, which requires reoperation. Undercorrected exotropia in children and adults usually does not resolve. If the angle is 15 PD or greater, reoperation must be considered.

REFERENCE

1. Kraft SP, Levin AV, Enzenauer RW. Unilateral surgery for exotropia with convergence weakness. *J Pediatr Ophthalmol Strabismus.* 1995;32:183-187.

SUGGESTED READINGS

Apt L, Call NB. Inferior oblique muscle recession. *Am J Ophthalmol.* 1978;85:95.

Biglan AW, Davis JS, Cheng KP, et al. Infantile exotropia. *J Pediatr Ophthalmol Strabismus.* 1996;33:79-84.

Choi DG, Rosenbaum AL. Medial rectus resections with adjustable suture for intermittent exotropia of the convergence insufficiency type. *J AAPOS.* 2001;5:13-17.

Davis D, McNeer KW, Spencer RF. Myectomy of the inferior oblique muscle. *Arch Ophthalmol.* 1986;104:855-858.

Hansen VC. Common pitfalls in measuring strabismic patients. *Am Orthopt J.* 1989;39:3.

Kirchen DG, Rosenbaum AL, Weiss S. Strabismus measurement errors on (prism) alternate cover test in amblyopes with eccentric fixation. *Binocular Vision Eye Muscle Q.* 1992;7:155.

Kushner BJ. Exotropic deviations: a functional classification and approach to treatment. *Am Orthopt J.* 1998;38:81-93.

Livir-Rallatos G, Gunton KB, Calhoun JH. Surgical results in large-angle exotropia. *J AAPOS.* 2000;6(2):77-80.

Moore S. The prognostic value of lateral gaze measurements in intermittent exotropia. *Am Orthop J.* 1969;19:69-71.

Nelson LB, Bacal DA, Burke MJ. An alternative approach to the surgical management of exotropia: the unilateral lateral rectus recession. *J Pediatr Ophthalmol Strabismus.* 1992;29:357-360.

Park J-H, Kim S-H. Clinical features and the risk factors of infantile exotropia recurrence. *Am J Ophthalmol.* 2010;150(4):464-467.e462.

Parks MM. The weakening surgical procedures for eliminating overaction of the inferior oblique muscle. *Am J Ophthalmol.* 1972;73:107.

Repka MX, Arnoldi KA. Lateral incomitance in exotropia: fact or artifact? *J Pediatr Ophthalmol Strabismus.* 1991;28:125-128; discussion 129-130.

Scattergood KD, Brown MH, Guyton DL. Artifacts introduced by spectacle lenses in the measurement of strabismic deviations. *Am J Ophthalmol.* 1983;96:439.

Stager DR, Parks MM. Inferior oblique weakening procedures. Effect on primary position horizontal alignment. *Arch Ophthalmol.* 1973;90:15-16.

Wang L, Nelson L. Outcome study of unilateral lateral rectus recession for small to moderate angle intermittent exotropia in children. *J Pediatr Ophthalmol Strabismus.* 2010;47:242-247.

4

Dissociated Vertical Deviation

Sepideh Tara Rousta, MD

There are few things more vexing to the pediatric ophthalmology team than *dissociated vertical deviation*, or DVD. The term *dissociated strabismus complex* has been preferred by some pediatric ophthalmologists because it refers to all the movements in the vertical, horizontal, and torsional axes. The condition is vexing because, having finally mastered how to measure and formulate a plan for the treatment of horizontal strabismus, one then uncovers the dreaded DVD.

A DVD occurs when an eye slowly elevates, extorts, and abducts during nonfixation or with visual inattention. Ophthalmology residents should take comfort in the fact that even among "experts," DVD remains an elusive and difficult ocular motor abnormality. Adding to the complexity of surgical treatment is the fact that DVD typically occurs in the setting of poor early binocular function. Often, it appears after congenital horizontal strabismus surgery, even when the horizontal outcome has been successful. Nevertheless, there are a variety of surgical approaches that can be used to treat DVD when it becomes manifest.

In his landmark article on DVD, Dr. David Guyton[1] elucidates the most likely underlying mechanisms with the use of dual-coil scleral search coils to measure eye movements 3-dimensionally. In the setting of early poor binocular function, fixating with the dominant eye or covering the weaker eye causes a cyclovertical latent nystagmus. The fixating eye actually intorts and depresses while the nonpreferred eye extorts and elevates. According

Nelson LB, Levin AV, eds.
The Wills Eye Strabismus Surgery Handbook (pp 25-32).
© 2015 Taylor & Francis Group.

to this research, these movements actually dampen the latent cyclovertical nystagmus. In Guyton's work with search coils, both eyes appear to be moving, vertically and torsionally, during DVD, even if only the nonfixating eye moves more visibly. This point is critical to understanding which muscles may be involved in DVD and therefore which surgical approaches should be favored.

A second possible etiology of DVD, discussed by Dr. Michael Brodsky,[2] is attributed to a dorsal left reflex that emerges when single binocular vision is prevented in infancy. If this hypothesis is correct, then patients should note a subjective sensation of tilt. Dr. Brodsky has shown that when alternate occlusion in patients with DVD is performed, many noted a tilt in the vertical plane. When occlusion of the fixating eye was performed in these patients, a vertical pencil position in the sagittal plane was perceived to be tilted, with the upper pole tilted toward the pull of the covered eye. This instantaneous tilt was quickly noted to be rotated back to the vertical plane.

In evaluating for DVD, it is important first to neutralize any horizontal deviations as well as any vertical deviation resembling a hypertropia. Hypertropias can be measured with the alternate cover test and have a typical quick vertical refixation movement of each eye, in accordance with Hering's law. DVD exhibits a slower, floating quality of the eye beneath the cover and a slower refixation movement when the eye is uncovered. If DVD is bilateral, each eye will drift in the upward direction when it is beneath the cover during alternate cover testing, thereby not appearing to follow Hering's law.

It is often very challenging to measure a DVD accurately. One method is to hold progressively higher base-down prisms over the eye behind the cover and check for refixation movements when the cover is removed. In poorly compliant children, the DVD may have to be estimated using a Krimsky test. Some place a neutral-density filter to blur one eye and elicit the DVD.

It is important to realize that DVD is often bilateral, although asymmetrical. Therefore, when one eye's vertical movements are neutralized, the other eye starts to float. Usually, bilateral base-down prisms are required simultaneously to obtain the best measurements. It is also paramount to test for inferior oblique overaction and to rate the degree on each side before devising a surgical plan for a case of DVD.

Case 1

Manifest DVD. OD = 15 in a 4-year-old. +4 RIO VA: OD 20/40, OS 20/30.

Surgeon 1: Anterior transposition of the RIO without myectomy and placed at 1 mm anterior and 2 mm lateral to the end of the inferior rectus insertion.

Surgeon 2: Prior to surgery, I would treat amblyopia OD. Then, I would anteriorize the RIO to the level of the RIR. I would warn the family that after surgery on the right eye, the child may develop an updrifting of the left eye and may require a similar procedure on the left eye.

Surgeon 3: RIO anterior transposition tightly bunched and 1 mm behind the RIR insertion.

Case 2

Same patient as Case 1 except +2 LIO.

Surgeon 1: Recess the superior rectus 5 mm.

Surgeon 2: Anteriorize the LIO to the level of the LIR and anteriorize the RIO 1 to 2 mm anterior to the RIR.

Surgeon 3: BIOAT with LIO tightly bunched 2 mm posterior to the insertion of the LIR and RIO 1 mm behind the RIR.

Case 3

Same patient as Case 1 except DVD OS = 10.

Surgeon 1: Anterior transposition of the RIO without myectomy and placed at 1 mm anterior and 2 mm lateral to the end of the RIR insertion; anterior transposition of the LIO without myectomy placed 2 mm lateral and parallel to the LIR insertion.

Surgeon 2: Anteriorize the LIO to the level or left inferior rectus and anteriorize the RIO 1 to 2 mm anterior to the RIR.

Surgeon 3: BIOAT as described for Case 2.

Case 4

DVD. OD = 18, OS = 12. + 1 IO OU.

Surgeon 1: Recess the superior rectus 6 mm OD with posterior fixation suture and recession of the superior rectus 4 mm OS with posterior fixation suture (Faden operation).

Surgeon 2: Anteriorize the LIO to the level of the LIR and anteriorize the RIO 1 to 2 mm anterior to the RIR.

Surgeon 3: BIOAT as described for Case 2.

Case 5

DVD. OS = 15 manifest. No IO OU overaction; VA, OU 20/25.

Surgeon 1: Recess the LSR 5 mm.

Surgeon 2: Recess the LSR 6 mm.

Surgeon 3: Recess the LSR 6 mm.

Case 6

RET = 20 minimal hyperopia OU. Manifest DVD. OD = 15. VA, OD 20/30, OS 20/25, +3 RIO.

Surgeon 1: Recess the RMR 6 mm and anterior transposition of the RIO without myectomy, placed at 1 mm anterior and 2 mm lateral to the end of the RIO insertion.

Surgeon 2: Resect the RLR 8 mm and anteriorize the RIO to the level of the RIR.

Surgeon 3: Resect the RLR 4 mm, RIOAT bunched tightly and 2 mm posterior to the RIR insertion.

Case 7

Same patient as Case 6 except no overacting RIO.

Surgeon 1: Recess the RMR 5 mm and recess the RSR 5 mm.

Surgeon 2: Resect the RLR 8 mm and recess the RSR 6 mm.

Surgeon 3: Resect the RLR 4 mm and recess the RSR 6 mm.

Case 8

Same patient as Case 6 except RXT = 20.

Surgeon 1: Recess the RLR 8 mm and anterior transposition of the RIO without myectomy and placed at 1 mm anterior and 2 mm lateral to the end of the RIR insertion.

Surgeon 2: Recess the LLR 8 mm and recess the RSR 6 mm.

Surgeon 3: Advance the RMR to original insertion. RIOAT bunched tightly and 2 mm posterior to the RIR insertion.

Case 9

+4 IO OU, DVD 10 OU; VA, OU 20/30.

Surgeon 1: Anterior transposition of the inferior oblique OU without myectomy.

Surgeon 2: Anteriorize the RIO and LIO to the level of the inferior rectus.

Surgeon 3: BIOAT bunched tightly at the BIR lateral insertion.

Case 10

DVD OU = 15. No IO OU overaction; VA, 20/30, OS 20/25.

Surgeon 1: Recess the superior rectus 5 mm plus posterior fixation suture OU.

Surgeon 2: Recess the RSR and the LSR 8 mm.

Surgeon 3: Recess the BSR 6 mm.

DISCUSSION

In planning the surgical approach to a DVD, certain information is critical. The vision is always important, since amblyopia should be treated prior to surgery, as is the case with any strabismus. Is the DVD manifest, occurring spontaneously and measurably before cover testing? The prism diopter measurement of the DVD itself must be determined, with special attention given to searching for a more subtle DVD movement in the other eye. Often, the DVD in the dominant eye is masked until the one in the nondominant eye is neutralized.

As mentioned previously, the function of each inferior oblique muscle should be tested with careful ductions and versions. Asymmetry in the level of possible inferior oblique overaction must be noted. If the inferior oblique overaction is rated +2 or higher, it must be dealt with surgically in the setting of a DVD, or a residual hypertropia may remain.

The major muscle surgeries advocated for DVD surgery aim to weaken elevation in one or both eyes. Superior rectus recession surgery alone or in combination with an inferior oblique weakening procedure is most common. Before surgery on the inferior oblique became more common, some surgeons did inferior rectus resections for DVDs.

When both elevators are weakened, there is always concern about causing a problematic elevation deficit. Because DVDs do not follow the same standard of dose response to vertical muscle surgery as ordinary hypertropias, the amount of surgery necessary to correct a DVD is greater than one would suppose.

In Case 1, the manifest DVD is unilateral in the weaker eye, and there is marked inferior oblique overaction. Unilateral surgery in such a case makes sense once the amblyopia has been treated, DVD in the other eye is ruled out, and the patient/family understands that there is still a possibility of a vertical deviation appearing in the other eye. Unilateral anterior transposition of the inferior oblique can be highly effective.[2] This procedure both weakens the overacting inferior oblique muscle and can use it to create an antielevation effect. It is important to note that the inferior oblique muscle, once isolated and cut at its insertion, should be bunched into a bundle rather than splayed out. Particular attention should be paid to the posterior fibers, making sure that they are incorporated into the bunching for full effect. This bundled inferior oblique is then transposed to the lateral edge of the inferior rectus muscle.

The antielevation effect of the transposed inferior oblique can be graded depending on where it is placed in relation to the inferior rectus insertion. A greater effect can be achieved by placing it 1 to 2 mm anterior to the border of the inferior rectus, whereas a lesser effect can be achieved by placing it a few millimeters posterior to the border of the inferior rectus.

As one can see from the responses, different surgeons advocate different degrees of anteriorization of the inferior oblique muscle. One must be cautious about this because this approach can lead to a symptomatic elevation deficit in primary position. There are cases in which the anteriorization has had to be surgically undone because of a restrictive hypotropia in the operated eye.

If a surgeon prefers to avoid anteriorization, there is another approach. Superior rectus recession can be done for the DVD amount measured, and the inferior oblique can simply be weakened by standard recession or myectomy depending on the degree of overaction.[3] This can prevent the pitfalls of the antielevation syndrome sometimes encountered with anteriorization. The downside to this approach is the need to operate on 2 muscles instead of one.

In Cases 4 through 6, in which a DVD exists in the setting of minimal (+1) or no inferior oblique overaction, most surgeons would perform unilateral or bilateral superior rectus recessions. Surgical dosing for how much to weaken the superior rectus varies. Because the DVD does not follow the same dose-response curve as standard hypertropia surgery, larger superior rectus recessions are necessary to prevent late recurrences. To adequately weaken the superior rectus in the setting of a DVD, recessions as large as 6 to 10 mm are preferred. Some surgeons will do a smaller recession of the superior rectus but will augment the weakening by adding a posterior fixation suture (Faden operation). The advantage of a Faden operation is that it weakens a muscle mainly in the direction of the muscle's primary action, in this case supraduction. The disadvantage is that the surgeon must place the sutures through the sclera fairly far back (12 to 15 mm), requiring good exposure and possibly risking perforation.

In performing large recessions of the superior rectus, one must be aware of the possibility of inducing changes to the palpebral fissure opening. It is important to dissect the superior rectus far back posteriorly, freeing it from attachments to the upper lid complex. The patient/parent should be warned about possible widening of the palpebral fissure opening. In addition, care should be taken not to injure or involve the superior oblique fibers as they pass beneath the posterior portion of the superior rectus muscle.

DVD often coexists in the setting of congenital esotropia and exotropia. Because early binocular development is poor in these patients, there is frequent recurrence of the horizontal deviation after initial early horizontal surgery. The DVD usually is not manifest until years after the horizontal deviation, typically between the ages of 3 and 5 years. Parents of infants undergoing early horizontal muscle surgery should be warned about the possibility, in some studies as high as 70%, of future vertical deviation.

As seen in Cases 6 through 8, DVD surgery can be done in conjunction with horizontal strabismus surgery. In Case 6, where both the horizontal deviation and the DVD are unilateral, anteriorizing the inferior oblique is particularly helpful because one can avoid injuring the anterior segment blood supply of the superior rectus muscle.

To summarize, a number of considerations come into play in planning surgery for a DVD. Although a DVD rarely causes diplopia, it can be disfiguring when frequently manifest. Once the decision to operate has been made, it is important to measure the DVD, determine its laterality, and decide if there is concurrent inferior oblique overaction. In the setting of combined DVD and significant inferior oblique overaction, many surgeons advocate anteriorization of the inferior oblique muscle. This can be done by bundling the fibers and transposing them just lateral to the inferior rectus insertion or 1 or 2 mm anterior or posterior to the insertion. Another preferred approach, especially in the setting of a larger DVD, is to perform a superior rectus recession in combination with inferior oblique recession or myectomy. When the DVD exists with minimal or no inferior oblique overaction, superior rectus recessions measuring 6 to 10 mm are preferred. Smaller superior rectus recessions can also be done in combination with a Faden posterior fixation suture. If the DVD is unilateral, one side can be done, but there is a chance that a DVD would then become manifest on the other side. For this reason, many surgeons will always recess both superior recti, sometimes asymmetrically.

REFERENCES

1. Guyton DL. Dissociated vertical deviation: etiology, mechanism, and associated phenomena. *J AAPOS.* 2000;4(3):131-144.
2. Brodsky MC. Dissociated vertical divergence: a righting reflex gone wrong. *Arch Ophthalmol.* 1999;117(9):1216-1222.
3. Varn MM, Saunders RA, Wilson ME. Combined bilateral superior rectus recession and inferior oblique muscle weakening for dissociated vertical deviation. *J AAPOS.* 1997;1(3):134-137.

SUGGESTED READINGS

Bothun ED, Summers CG. Unilateral inferior oblique anterior transposition for dissociated vertical deviation. *J AAPOS.* 2004;8(3):259-263.

Nabie R, Anvari F, Azadeh M, Ameri A, Jafari A. Evaluation of the effectiveness of anterior transposition of the inferior oblique muscle in dissociated vertical deviation with or without inferior oblique overaction. *J Pediatr Ophthalmol Strabismus.* 2007;44:158-162.

5

Cranial Nerve Palsies

Mary O'Hara, MD

The surgical approach to the patient with cranial nerve palsy can vary greatly from case to case and surgeon to surgeon. In planning surgery, one must consider specific motility deficits, the age and functionality of the patient, and his or her postsurgical expectations. The individual "style" of the surgeon also comes into play. Specific surgical doses vary as a result of nuances in surgical technique. Because of these factors, there is no one-size-fits-all approach.

There are unifying principles that help to guide us. An accurate history will help to establish whether the strabismus is congenital or acquired. Sensory adaptations are important in planning for diplopia avoidance; strabismus caused by congenital cranial nerve palsy with sensory adaptations may warrant a different surgical approach from an identical cranial nerve palsy in a patient with prior fusion who is now diplopic because of an acute cranial nerve palsy. Attention to nonstrabismic aspects of the motility examination is also important; correction of head turns and torsion must be incorporated into the surgical plan. Timing for the repair of associated problems such as ptosis must also be part of the planning.

In acute-onset cranial nerve palsy, a workup of the underlying cause of the palsy is necessary. A waiting period before surgery is also warranted because there may be recovery of muscle function over time. During this observational period for patients with acute sixth-nerve palsies, botulinum toxin injected into the ipsilateral medial rectus will paralyze the muscle and

Nelson LB, Levin AV, eds.
The Wills Eye Strabismus Surgery Handbook (pp 33-43).
© 2015 Taylor & Francis Group.

hopefully prevent secondary contracture. Most surgeons defer strabismus surgery for 6 to 12 months after the onset of strabismus due to cranial nerve palsy. Many counsel the patient that multiple strabismus surgeries may be required or describe the process as a staged procedure. Since full normal motility and orthotropia in all fields of gaze cannot usually be restored, the surgeon must listen to the patient to determine which approach would afford the patient best function in his or her daily life.

Case 1

CN III palsy: LXT = 70. Inability to elevate, depress, or adduct OS even to the midline.

Surgeon 1: Disinsert the LLR by placing on 6-0 nonabsorbable suture, passing the suture 10 mm posterior to the insertion, and then hanging back and being sure to push the muscle through Tenon's fascia. Then, fixate the globe to the nasal orbital wall by passing a polypropylene suture adjacent to the LMR and fixing to the periosteum of the nasal wall.

Surgeon 2: Recess the LLR 16 mm.

Surgeon 3: First, I would do forced ductions under anesthesia. If normal, I would recess the LLR 12 mm and then resect the LMR 12 mm and place the LMR on an adjustable suture, which could then be adjusted postoperatively as necessary. If the forced ductions were abnormal, I would identify what the restriction was and change the procedure as necessary.

Case 2

CN III palsy: LXT = 70. LHT = 15. Inability to elevate, depress, or adduct OS even to the midline.

Surgeon 1: Fix XT as in Case 1. With the LSO as the only functional vertically active muscle, no surgery for the left hypertropia at this time.

Surgeon 2: Recess the LLR 16 mm and anterior transposition of the LIO temporal and parallel to the insertion of the LIR. No myectomy of the LIO.

Surgeon 3: Same as in Case 1. After getting the eye as close to alignment in the primary position, I would reevaluate the HT, which might be gone. If it is still present, I would wait 6 months and then recess the LSR as needed.

Case 3

Partial CN III palsy: LXT = 35. Able to adduct OS just beyond the midline.

Surgeon 1: Resect the LMR 5 mm and recess the LLR 10 mm with the LLR on an adjustable suture.

Surgeon 2: Recess the LLR 8 mm and resect the LMR 5.5 mm.

Surgeon 3: If this were an adult, I would use topical anesthesia. I would do forced ductions and then recess the LLR 7 mm and resect the LMR 7 mm. I would then reevaluate this postoperatively. If this were a child, I would do the forced ductions and recess the LLR 10 mm and reevaluate postoperatively.

Case 4

CN III palsy with pupil sparing: 8-month-old boy born with ptosis and exotropia OD. CNS workup negative. RSR, RIR, RMR –3 to –4 underaction with ptosis 4 mm, intorsion intact. RXT = 30, RhypoT = 10.

What is the first operation you would do?

What would you then do to treat residual XT and hypotropia?

Special considerations regarding ptosis repair?

What expectations of the eventual outcome would you communicate to the parents?

Surgeon 1: What is the first operation you would do? Recess the RLR 10 mm.

What would you then do to treat residual XT and hypotropia? Disinsert the RSO and attach the RSO adjacent to the RMR.

Special considerations regarding ptosis repair? Frontalis sling will be required. Ptosis must be treated early, as treatment for amblyopia must be aggressive.

What expectations of the eventual outcome would you communicate to the parents? Very low chance for binocularity and high risk of amblyopia. I would try to get the right eye straight in primary position if possible. If face turn develops, some binocularity has been achieved with risk of amblyopia reduced. Monitoring of vision is vital. Lids will always be asymmetric.

Surgeon 2: What is the first operation you would do? Recess the RLR 10 mm.

What would you then do to treat residual XT and hypotropia? Six months later, resect the RMR and recess the RIR 3.5 mm.

Special considerations regarding ptosis repair? Frontalis suspension to the right upper eyelid performed following the strabismus surgery. I would leave the lid undercorrected because of concern of postoperative corneal dryness.

What expectations of the eventual outcome would you communicate to the parents? I would tell the parents that it is impossible to make the paralyzed muscles normal and would attempt to get the eyes as straight as possible in the primary position.

Surgeon 3: What is the first operation you would do? I would do FD, which would help to determine whether restriction was present; then recess the RLR 9 mm and resect the RMR 8 mm.

What would you then do to treat residual XT and hypotropia? Wait 6 months, then evaluate the hypotropia and recess the RIR 4 mm for the hypotropia. Might also have to reresect the RMR.

Special considerations regarding ptosis repair? I would solve the vertical strabismus first and then do a frontalis sling.

What expectations of the eventual outcome would you communicate to the parents? The objective is to align the eyes as straight as possible in the primary position. It is not possible to have normal rotations after surgery.

Case 5

CN IV palsy: 6-month-old girl with a 15-degree right head tilt. Approximate LHT = 15, no overaction LIO.

Surgeon 1: LSO tendon tuck until tight.

Surgeon 2: LSO tendon tuck.

Surgeon 3: I would evaluate the hypertropia as well as possible in all positions of gaze. There is an LHT of 15 PD in the primary, so I would recess the LSR 4 mm and see what the results were. If there was a residual LHT, I would favor recessing the RIR.

Case 6

CN IV palsy: left head tilt = 10 degrees. RHT = 18. RHT = 24 in left gaze, RHT = 19 in right gaze. +4 RIO.

Surgeon 1: Recess the RIO without myectomy and slight anteriorization 3 mm posterior to the RIR.

Surgeon 2: Recess the RIO 14 mm from the RIR insertion. No myectomy.

Surgeon 3: Forced ductions. Because there is RHT in the primary position that is greater in left gaze and an overacting RIO, I would sever the RIO from the sclera. I would then find the lateral edge of the RIR insertion. I would reattach the RIO 2 mm temporal and 3 mm posterior to this edge. A later recession of the LIR might be needed.

Case 7

CN IV palsy: right head tilt = 10 degrees. LHT = 25. LHT = 30 in right gaze, LHT = 25 in left gaze. +4 LIO.

Surgeon 1: Standard LIO recession without myectomy. Recess the LSR 4 mm.

Surgeon 2: Recess the LIO 14 mm from the left inferior rectus insertion. No myectomy. Recess the LSR 3 mm.

Surgeon 3: There is LHT of 25 PD in the primary position and overaction of the LIO. I would sever the LIO tendon from the sclera and reattach it to the sclera as described in Case 6. Most likely, there will be a residual LHT. I would wait 6 weeks. If there is a residual LHT, I would recess the RIR 3 to 4 mm, depending on the amount of the HT.

Case 8

CN IV palsy: long-standing LHT = 25 comitant in right and left gaze, right head tilt = 10 degrees. +4 LIO.

Surgeon 1: Standard LIO recession without myectomy. Recess the LSR 4 mm.

Surgeon 2: Recess the LIO 14 mm from the LIR insertion. No myectomy. Recess the LSR 3 mm.

Surgeon 3: Recess the LIO and do a later recession of the RIR. My standard weakening procedure on the IO is to sever it from the sclera and reattach it just temporal and posterior to the lateral border of the IR. This is a 14-mm recession as previously described. I never do a myectomy on the IO.

Case 9

CN IV palsy: closed head trauma 1 year earlier. Complaining of tilting of objects viewed. RHT = 2.12-degree exocyclotorsion.

Surgeon 1: RSO Harada-Ito placed at the superior border of the lateral rectus muscle 8 mm posterior to its insertion.

Surgeon 2: Bilateral Harada-Ito procedure performed by placing the anterior fibers of each superior oblique muscle inferior and approximately 8 mm posterior of the lateral rectus muscle of each eye.

Surgeon 3: I would perform a Harada-Ito procedure. I would operate the SO between the trochlea and the SR. I would split its tendon into anterior and posterior halves. I would then sever the anterior half from the sclera and reattach it to the sclera 8 mm posterior and inferior to the LR insertion.

Case 10

CN VI palsy: closed head trauma 1 year earlier. Complaints of horizontal diplopia. Left face turn = 15 degrees. LET = 50. Unable to abduct OS past the midline. Elevation, depression, and adduction OS normal.

Surgeon 1: LSR transposition to the superior border of the LLR augmented with posterior fixation suture of LLR at 8 mm from insertion.

Surgeon 2: Recess the LMR 15 mm.

Surgeon 3: If the patient were an adult I would use topical anesthesia and do forced ductions. If the eye could not be moved temporally, I would sever the MR from the sclera and repeat the forced ductions. If the forced ductions were then normal, I would recess the MR 7 mm and stop. I would then reevaluate the problem postoperatively. If the forced ductions were normal from the beginning and no restriction were present, I would recess the MR 9 mm and resect the LR 14 mm. If the patient were a child, I would use general anesthesia and perform forced ductions. If they were normal, I would recess the MR 9 mm and resect the LR 14 mm.

Case 11

CN VI palsy: intracranial aneurysm repaired 6 months earlier. Immediately after repair, diplopia noted. Now patient has RET = 75, is unable to abduct OD past the midline. Elevation, depression, and adduction normal OD.

Surgeon 1: RSR transposition to the superior border of the RLR augmented with fixation suture to the LLR 8 mm posterior to its insertion.

Surgeon 2: Recess the RMR 15 mm. May need Jensen procedure as a later surgery.

Surgeon 3: Topical anesthesia. Is the MR tight? Recess the RMR 9 mm and resect the RLR 14 mm.

Case 12

CN VI palsy: closed head trauma 2 years earlier, onset of diplopia noted immediately. RET = 30. Able to abduct OD just beyond the midline. Elevation, depression, and adduction OD normal.

Surgeon 1: Forced duction. If the RMR is tight, consider botulinum toxin to the RMR and remeasure. Once the effect of the botulinum toxin is gone (8 to 10 weeks), then recess the RMR 4.5 mm and resect the RLR 8 mm if still 30 PD.

Surgeon 2: Recess the RMR 7 mm.

Surgeon 3: In an adult, I would use topical anesthesia and perform forced ductions. If they were normal, I would recess the MR 6 mm and resect the LR 10 mm. If the forced ductions were positive, I would sever the MR from the sclera and repeat the forced ductions. If the forced ductions were then normal, it would tell me that the MR was tight. I would then recess the MR 7 mm and resect the LR 12 mm. If the patient were a child, I would do the forced ductions before and during the operation, as noted in regard to the adult. I would use the same guidelines for the amount of surgery as in the adult.

Case 13

Bilateral CN VI palsy: removal of a benign brain tumor 1 year earlier. Diplopia noted immediately. ET = 90. Unable to abduct either eye beyond the midline. Elevation, depression, and adduction OU normal.

Surgeon 1: Staged procedure with transposition of each SR to the respective LR with augmentation suture to LR 8 mm posterior to insertion. Wait 6 weeks for effect. Then, recess the BMR for residual ET.

Surgeon 2: Recess the MR OU 15 mm.

Surgeon 3: If the patient were a child, I would do forced ductions under anesthesia to determine if there were any tightness of the medial rectus muscles. I would then recess the MR of the nondominant eye 9 mm and resect the LR 14 mm. The amount of surgery would not vary, regardless of whether the forced ductions were positive. If the patient were an adult, I would favor topical anesthesia and perform forced ductions before and during the operation, as with a child. I would then recess the MR 9 mm and resect the LR 14 mm. In both adults and children, there would be the likelihood of a residual ET after surgery. The results of that surgery would then give me a better idea of how to adjust the amount of surgery on the other eye.

Discussion

The varying presentations and surgical options for the treatment of motility deficits secondary to cranial nerve palsies challenge the strabismus surgeon. The 3 surgeons in this chapter share their approaches to these complex problems. Although their individual surgical plans vary, certain aspects of their plans are universally applied.

Two tests that may assist the surgeon in the planning stage are forced duction and active forced generation. In the forced-duction test, the anesthetized eye is mechanically moved into various positions of gaze to detect any resistance to passive movement. Resistance to passive movement is considered a positive test. The active forced-generation test is helpful in determining the residual function of paretic muscles. With the eye stabilized with forceps, the patient is asked to move the eye in the opposite direction. If the examiner detects a tug on the forceps, some residual function of the involved eye exists.

The first set of cases (1 through 4) deals with variations on the theme of third-nerve palsy. Strabismus from third-nerve palsy can be among the most surgically challenging cases that a strabismus surgeon will encounter. Oculomotor palsies can be complete or partial. The motility pattern may be confounded by aberrant regeneration. It is not unusual, then, that surgical approaches will vary.[1,2] All of the cases presented had some degree of incomitant exotropia. All 3 surgeons said that they would employ a lateral rectus weakening procedure to address the exotropia. In certain cases, an adjustable suture can be used to fine tune alignment. Case 1 is a complete third-nerve palsy, whereas Case 2 is a complete third-nerve palsy with hypertropia. Some surgeons would address the hypertropia immediately, whereas others would choose a staged approach. Case 3 is a partial third-nerve palsy with some medial rectus function. A recess/resect procedure would be chosen more commonly in this scenario. A congenital pupil-sparing third-nerve palsy with associated ptosis (Case 4) elicited several surgical approaches. All 3 surgeons would address the horizontal deviation first and then reserve treatment of the hypotropia for a second surgery. One surgeon proposed transposition of the superior oblique to the superior medial rectus insertion to address the vertical deviation and strengthen adduction, while her colleagues proposed surgery on a vertical muscle to address the vertical component combined with additional medial rectus surgery to address the adduction deficit. All the surgeons recommended ptosis surgery after strabismus surgery. Caution is warranted and a conservative degree of elevation is advised to prevent corneal compromise.

The second set of cases (5 to 9) highlights various presentations of fourth-nerve palsy. The surgical approach suggested was more uniform with this group of cases, reflecting favorable treatment options that have been shown to have good outcomes.[3] Case 6 represents a fourth-nerve palsy with a moderate degree of hypertropia and inferior oblique overaction. All 3 surgeons would address the inferior oblique in their initial surgery. This reflects the importance of lateral incomitance in surgical planning. When, in Case 5, a similar hypertropia was present without inferior oblique overaction, none of the surgeons would have elected to operate on the inferior oblique. Two of them recommended a superior oblique tuck, whereas one would opt for a wait-and-see approach. The larger hypertropia in primary position in Case 7 prompted the addition of surgery on a second cyclovertical extraocular muscle. Long-standing strabismus secondary to cranial nerve palsies tends to become more comitant over time, a condition referred to as *spread of comitance*. Case 8 presented a long-standing fourth-nerve palsy. The spread of comitance seen in this case would not have altered the surgical plans. Case 9 demonstrates a fourth-nerve palsy with a functional deficit that was primarily excyclotorsion. All 3 surgeons would have elected to address the excyclotorsion with a Harada-Ito procedure, a superior oblique surgery that decreases excyclotorsion without significantly affecting the vertical alignment.

The final set of cases presents different manifestations of sixth-nerve palsy. Surgical plans varied by surgeon. One surgeon would opt for botulinum toxin as an adjunct to surgery.[4] Cases 10 and 11 are complete sixth-nerve palsies with different etiologies. Case 10 demonstrates a complete traumatic sixth-nerve palsy that persisted for 1 year. Case 11 is a complete sixth-nerve palsy that persisted for 6 months after neurological lesion. Etiology did not alter the recommended surgical approach to the strabismus, although the surgical approaches varied from surgeon to surgeon. Most surgeons would employ some form of transposition procedure when addressing a complete sixth-nerve palsy. The risk of anterior segment necrosis must be considered in this surgical approach, since 4 of the 7 anterior ciliary arteries would be compromised with full transposition surgery. One surgeon would use a full transposition procedure as the initial approach to the larger-angle esotropia. The other 2 surgeons would address the horizontal muscles initially. One proposes a Jenson transposition as a possible second-stage procedure, preserving the vertical blood supply to the anterior segment of the eye. When, in Case 12, the sixth-nerve palsy was partial and some medial rectus function was present, all 3 surgeons proposed horizontal muscle surgery. One recommended a trial of botulinum toxin to the medial rectus muscle preoperatively to determine the dose of surgery. The profound esotropia due to bilateral sixth-nerve palsies present in Case 13 resulted in different proposed surgical approaches. One surgeon again chose to address the bilateral complete sixth-nerve palsy with transposition procedures while the others chose horizontal surgery.

Several adjuncts to surgery can be employed in the surgical plan. Forced ductions and force generation can be employed to identify specific extraocular muscle deficits in designing the surgical plan. In general, strabismus surgeons prefer to reduce restriction and avoid relying on very paretic muscles to generate alignment forces. Botulinum toxin can be used diagnostically and therapeutically. In some cases, an antagonist muscle can be paralyzed as part of the surgical plan. In others, botulinum toxin can be used to paralyze an antagonist muscle preoperatively to determine the degree of function of a palsied muscle. Prism adaptation testing may better refine the operative dose of strabismus surgery. Neuroimaging can also be helpful in guiding strabismus surgery. Cranial nerve palsies after trauma may include associated orbital or muscular changes that would alter the strabismus surgeon's plan.

Preoperative counseling must be emphasized. In treating cranial nerve palsies, it is critically important to outline realistic expectations and goals for the patient. In most cases, full ductions and versions are not attainable. Surgery may have to be staged. Patients must be aware that several surgeries may be necessary to achieve realistic goals. One must also consider the possibility that multiple cranial nerve palsies may be present. It is important to address patient expectations in this context as well. Many patients believe that the realignment of an eye will restore its vision. This mistaken idea must be addressed preoperatively. Expectations for diplopia relief must also be outlined preoperatively. A successful outcome may be possible only in primary and reading positions, and this should be the target. The patient may still need prism in spectacles after strabismus surgery to treat residual diplopia. In operating on multiple muscles, there may be a risk of anterior segment ischemia. The surgeons staged certain surgeries and designed surgical plans that did not remove more than 2 rectus muscles at a time in a given eye.

The surgical correction of motility defects secondary to cranial nerve palsies requires an individualized approach. Various procedures can be effective in restoring at least partial function. There is no wrong answer in planning surgery. The surgical goal is to plan an operation or operations that optimize the individual patient's outcome.

REFERENCES

1. Yonghong J, Kanxing Z, Wei L, Xiao W, Jinghui W, Fanghua Z. Surgical management of large-angle incomitant strabismus in patients with oculomotor nerve palsy. *J AAPOS*. 2008;12(1):49-53.

2. Flanders M, Hasan J, Al-Mujaini A. Partial third nerve palsy: clinical characteristics and surgical management. *Can J Ophthalmol*. 2012;47(3):321-325.

3. Bagheri A, Fallahi M, Abrishami M, Salour H, Aletaha M. Clinical features and outcomes of treatment for fourth nerve palsy. *J Ophthalmol Vision Res*. 2010;5(1):27-31.

4. Bagheri A, Babsharif B, Abrishami M, Salour H, Aletaha M. Outcomes of surgical and non-surgical treatment for sixth nerve palsy. *J Ophthalmol Vision Res*. 2010;5(1):32-37.

6

Strabismus Syndromes

Mark A. Steele, MD

There are a number of treatment possibilities for the variety of strabismus syndromes. This chapter addresses congenital cranial dysinnervation disorders, including DRS, Möbius syndrome, CFEOM, and DEP. The restrictive Brown syndrome is also discussed, as is the rare syndrome of cyclic esotropia.

The significant majority of patients presenting with these syndromes will exhibit incomitant strabismic deviations. As a result, affected individuals will frequently maintain an anomalous compensatory head posture to place their eyes in the gaze position where the ocular alignment is best and binocular vision is achieved. Binocularity is a very important prompt, even in small infants, to assume a compensatory head posture.

The treatment strategy for these patients with complex strabismus is to strive to align the eyes in primary gaze, afford the broadest field of single binocular vision possible, and alleviate the compensatory anomalous head position. A thorough preoperative examination including measurement of the strabismic angle in all gaze positions, including right and left tilt, is essential for properly planning restorative surgery. The results of intraoperative forced duction testing may alter the surgical plan, as recessions of restricted extraocular muscles and relief of other extraocular restrictions that may be present will often help to secure an optimal postsurgical outcome.

Nelson LB, Levin AV, eds.
The Wills Eye Strabismus Surgery Handbook (pp 45-55).
© 2015 Taylor & Francis Group.

Case 1

Type I DRS OS. Left face turn = 25 degrees. ET = 25 PD in primary position. No abduction OS past midline.

Surgeon 1: Recess the LMR 6 mm.

Surgeon 2: Recess the LMR 6 mm.

Surgeon 3: Is the ET of 25 the primary or secondary deviation? If it is the primary deviation (on which such surgery should be based), I would recess the LMR 6 mm. If the adduction of the left eye is poor, there is a risk that a large medial rectus recession would result in synergistic divergence.

Case 2

Same patient as Case 1 with a large leash effect upward on attempted adduction OS.

Surgeon 1: Recess the LMR 6 mm and Y-split the LLR.

Surgeon 2: Recess the LMR 6 mm. Anterior transposition of the LIO to the temporal border of the LIR insertion.

Surgeon 3: Same as Case 1 and Y-split the LLR.

Case 3

Type II DRS OS with a right face turn of 25 degrees. XT = 20 PD in primary position. No adduction OS past midline.

Surgeon 1: Recess the LLR 8 mm.

Surgeon 2: Recess the LLR 8 mm.

Surgeon 3: Recess the LLR 8 mm.

Case 4

Type I DRS OU. Alternating face turn with ET = 25 PD in primary position.

Surgeon 1: Recess the BMR 4 mm.

Surgeon 2: Recess either MR 6 mm.

Surgeon 3: Recess the BMR 4 mm.

Case 5

Möbius syndrome with bilateral sixth- and seventh-nerve palsies.
ET = 65 PD. Unable to abduct OU beyond the midline.

Surgeon 1: Transpose the SR and IR to the LR insertion OU.

Surgeon 2: Recess the BMR 7 mm.

Surgeon 3: Recess the BMR 6.5 mm.

Case 6

A 5-year-old boy with ET = 35 PD for several years with cycloplegic
refraction +0.50 OU. Parents state ET is not always present. Examination
1 week later shows orthophoria. Return visit the next day, ET = 35 PD. Cyclic
esotropia.

Surgeon 1: Recess the BMR 5 mm.

Surgeon 2: Recess 1 MR 7 mm of nondominant eye.

Surgeon 3: Recess the BMR 5 mm.

Case 7

DEP OD with right hypotropia 25 PD. Unable to elevate OD above the
midline. With OD fixation in primary position, the pseudoptosis disap-
pears.

Surgeon 1: Full-tendon transposition of the RMR and RLR to the RSR
insertion (Knapp procedure).

Surgeon 2: Full-tendon transposition of the RMR and RLR to the RSR
insertion (Knapp procedure).

Surgeon 3: Forced duction at time of surgery would determine if patient
has DEP or restricted IR. If forced duction negative, would perform
Knapp procedure OD.

Case 8

Same patient as Case 7 but right hypotropia is 15 PD.

Surgeon 1: Half-tendon transposition of the RMR and RLR to the RSR
insertion.

Surgeon 2: Recess the RIR 5 mm.

Surgeon 3: Recess the RIR 4 mm.

Case 9

Left face turn = 10 degrees. Right hypotropia is 10 PD in primary position. Unable to elevate OD in the adduction position; elevation improves in the straight-up and abducting positions. Brown syndrome.

Surgeon 1: RSO 6-mm tendon expander using silicone band.

Surgeon 2: Tenotomy RSO and recess RIO 14 mm.

Surgeon 3: Check forced ductions at time of surgery. If Brown syndrome is confirmed with positive forced ductions, then tenotomy of the RSO and recess the RIO 10 mm; if forced ductions negative, then recess the LSR 3 mm.

Case 10

A 5-year-old girl underwent insertion of a 7-mm silicone expander by another surgeon into her left superior oblique tendon for a left Brown syndrome. Her Brown syndrome is now worse with a head tilt and a left hypotropia in primary position of 10 PD.

What if she has a left hypotropia of 20 PD?

Surgeon 1: If forced ductions positive, then release of scarring around silicone expander. May need to remove expander, leaving tenotomy, and recess the LIO 14 mm. Same plan for 20 PD left hypotropia, but may need staged second procedure for any residual vertical strabismus. If forced ductions negative, then recess the RSR 3 mm for 10 PD and 6 mm for 20 PD.

Surgeon 2: For left hypotropia of 10 PD, recess the LIR 3.5 mm. For left hypotropia of 20 PD, recess the LIR 7 mm.

Surgeon 3: Remove silicone expander if 10 PD or 20 PD hypotropia.

Case 11

Congenital fibrosis syndrome OU in a 3-year-old boy. Maintains a 25-degree chin-up position. Both eyes can elevate just to the midline. Orthophoria in downgaze.

Surgeon 1: Confirm diagnosis with forced ductions. Recess the BIR 7 mm or BIR tenotomy OU depending on tightness. If very restricted, then BIR tenotomy.

Surgeon 2: Recess the BIR 10 mm.

Surgeon 3: Confirm diagnosis with forced duction. BIR tenotomy.

Case 12

Congenital fibrosis OD in a 4-year-old with a right hypotropia 30 PD and a chin-up position of 20 degrees.

Surgeon 1: Recess the RIR 7 mm. Consider LSR recess as subsequent procedure if needed.

Surgeon 2: Recess the RIR 10 mm.

Surgeon 3: Recess the RIR 6 mm.

Discussion

Duane Retraction Syndrome

DRS is a CCDD caused by nuclear or cranial nerve VI dysgenesis and secondary misinnervation by cranial nerve III, resulting in cocontraction of the medial and lateral recti in adduction (or, in the case of DRS types II and III, attempted adduction). As a result, there is retraction of the globe and narrowing of the interpalpebral fissure in adduction. Many patients with DRS do not require any intervention because they have straight eyes and binocular vision in primary gaze and therefore no anomalous head position. There is a subset of type I DRS with significant hyperopia with esotropia in primary gaze that can be partially or completely neutralized with eyeglasses alone. The surgical indications for patients with DRS include significant strabismus in primary gaze, presence of an anomalous head position, significant upshooting or downshooting of the eye in adduction, or marked narrowing of the interpalpebral fissure and globe retraction in adduction.

Neutralization of the strabismic deviation in primary gaze will prompt resolution of the anomalous head posture. In type I DRS, the typical deviation in primary gaze is an esotropia; in type II, an exotropia is generally seen. The consensus of opinion (as illustrated in the responses to Cases 1, 3, and 4) is to recess the appropriate ipsilateral rectus muscle. In treating type I DRS, others have proposed a full tendon superior rectus temporal transposition with or without the ipsilateral medial rectus recession. Occasionally, for larger deviations in primary gaze, additional horizontal rectus recessions may be required on the contralateral eye. Rectus muscle resections are generally avoided in DRS to avoid worsening globe retraction in adduction.

The upshooting and/or downshooting of the involved eye in adduction appears to not be specifically due to the cocontraction of the rectus muscles but rather to a mechanical effect. When the eye is adducting or attempting to adduct against a cocontracting lateral rectus, a mechanical "side slippage" of the globe may appear as an overelevation or overdepression of the globe. As indicated in responses to Case 2, this is often very well treated with a longitudinal Y-split of the ipsilateral lateral rectus muscle. This will serve to stabilize the globe in adduction, thus diminishing the anomalous upshooting or downshooting. Alternatively, a balanced simultaneous recession of the medial and lateral rectus muscles of the involved eye will also serve to diminish upshooting or downshooting in adduction and, in addition, diminish globe retraction and narrowing of the interpalpebral fissure in adduction. A balanced recession of the horizontal recti would not change the ocular alignment in primary gaze. For example, a 6-mm recession of the medial rectus combined with a 9-mm recession of the lateral rectus would diminish any upshoots or downshoots in adduction and diminish globe retraction without inducing a strabismus in primary gaze.

Möbius Syndrome

This rare congenital syndrome is characterized by facial diplegia and lateral gaze palsy. Aside from the typically bilateral palsies of cranial nerves VI and VII, other cranial nerve palsies and limb anomalies may be present. This disorder is believed to be a CCDD, likely due to mutations in genes relevant to axonal genesis and sprouting. Others have postulated a role for embryonic vascular insufficiency leading to ischemia of the cranial nerve nuclei.

Patients with Möbius syndrome will typically have a significant esotropia in primary gaze arising from the palsy of cranial nerve VI, as in Case 5. A variety of surgical approaches to correcting this form of strabismus have been reported, with variable outcomes. Generally, it is best to treat the strabismus in Möbius syndrome in the same way that a patient with a palsy of cranial nerve VI would be treated. Performing only medial rectus recessions is often not adequate in this setting. Depending on the magnitude of the esotropia and the results of intraoperative forced duction testing, a superior and inferior vertical rectus transposition with or without a medial rectus recession is often required. If there is significant forced duction positivity in abduction, the medial rectus would have to be recessed. A 7-mm recession of the medial rectus would alleviate approximately 35 PD of esotropia. If more effect were required, full-tendon transposition and Jensen transposition (where the lateral halves of the longitudinally split vertical recti are joined at the globe equator to the corresponding split halves of the lateral rectus) have been used successfully for these patients to create more abducting forces. The benefit of the Jensen procedure is the preservation of the vertical rectus contribution to the anterior ciliary circulation, which becomes especially important if a simultaneous medial rectus recession is performed. If forced duction testing is negative, only vertical rectus transpositions may be required.

Cyclic Esotropia

This peculiar and rare form of strabismus is characterized by alternating periods of esotropia and orthophoria as indicated in Case 6. The periodic cycles may occur over 1 or 2 days or more. On the days of orthophoria, there is no latent esodeviation. Curiously, surgical correction for the full convergent strabismic angle present on esotropic days will afford postoperative orthophoria on all days.

Brown Syndrome

Patients with Brown syndrome have a restriction of the SO tendon at its trochlear cartilage. This is typically congenital and generally resolves spontaneously and completely within the second decade of life. There are less common acquired forms that follow trauma or are secondary to inflammatory disease.

As illustrated in Case 9, the hallmark clinical presentation is an elevation deficit in adduction. The diminishing vertical duction deficit as the eye moves from adduction to abduction helps differentiate Brown syndrome from double elevator palsy or CFEOM. Although not large, there is often some overdepression in adduction (superior oblique overaction). An exotropia in upgaze is also common. Although positive intraoperative forced duction testing confirms the diagnosis of Brown syndrome, there are clinical observations that can help differentiate this syndrome from an isolated ipsilateral IO palsy. An IO palsy will have the characteristic pattern with the Parks-Bielschowsky 3-step test. For example, a left IO palsy will present with a right hypertropia worse in right gaze and right tilt. Patients with IO palsy will often present with ipsilateral compensatory head tilt, while those with Brown syndrome will frequently assume a chin-up or a contralateral face turn head posture. Unlike patients with Brown syndrome, those with IO palsy will have no exotropia in upgaze. Rather, an A pattern deviation may be present. The observation of fundus intorsion is not helpful in differentiating Brown syndrome and IO palsy because it may be present in either disorder.

The indications for surgical intervention in a child with congenital Brown syndrome include the presence of strabismus in primary gaze with or without an anomalous compensatory chin-up or face-turn head posture. Given the relatively higher reoperation rate and the transient nature of congenital Brown syndrome, surgery must be considered only if there is a significant vertical strabismus in primary gaze. The presence of a complete elevation deficiency in adduction is in itself not an indication for surgery. Many surgical techniques for alleviating the restriction of the SO tendon have been proposed, with mixed results. SO tenectomy or tenotomy with or without a simultaneous ipsilateral IO weakening (to thwart the possibility of an iatrogenic SO palsy) are most commonly performed. SO recession or SO weakening via a "Z tenotomy" has been described, as has insertion of an intratendon silicone spacer or nonabsorbable "chicken suture" that bridges the space between the cut tendon edges.

One reasonable approach to a patient with Brown syndrome confirmed by forced duction testing and who requires surgery is to tailor the procedure on the basis of the degree of hypotropia in primary gaze. For a small hypotropia of 6 PD or less, a posterior seven-eighths tenectomy of the SO will often work well. For 7 to 15 PD, an SO tenectomy with simultaneous IO weakening is a reasonable approach. For larger hypotropias, an SO tenectomy alone is preferred. Of course, informing the patient and/or guardian of the possibility that the child might require more than one surgical procedure is advisable. A silicone band spacer or nonabsorbable chicken suture may not sufficiently correct the hypotropia. Case 10 illustrates how these foreign materials can also lead to excessive scar formation and inflammation and potential extrusion of the silicone.

Double Elevator Palsy

DEP may be better termed *monocular elevation deficiency* to highlight the multiple etiologies of this ocular motility disturbance. True DEP is congenital and occurs sporadically. The causes include a supranuclear defect appearing clinically as palsy of the SR and IO. Other causes of monocular elevation deficiency include primary SR paresis, primary IR restriction, and IR restriction secondary to SR paresis. In patients with supranuclear DEP, supraduction may be intact in eliciting a Bell's response. The hallmark finding of DEP is an inability to elevate the eye from primary gaze, abduction, and adduction. Approximately 50% of patients with DEP have a true ipsilateral upper lid ptosis, to be distinguished from a pseudoptosis in the hypotropic eye.

For patients with DEP who demonstrate a significant vertical strabismus in primary gaze with or without an anomalous compensatory chin-up head posture, eye muscle surgery is indicated. Surgical management should start with an intraoperative forced duction test. Should there be restriction in elevation, an IR recession (range, 4 to 8 mm) may be considered. If forced duction testing is negative, as in Case 7, then all of our surgeons recommended a Knapp procedure. This involves superiorly transposing the horizontal rectus tendons to lie beside the superior rectus insertion. The Knapp procedure will correct anywhere from 20 to 35 PD of hypotropia. Should a significant hypotropia persist after a Knapp procedure, an IR recession may be needed. For a patient with DEP presenting with a smaller hypotropia (less than 20 PD), as exemplified in Case 8, and no restriction of the IR, either an IR recession alone or a superior transposition of the superior halves of the horizontal recti rather than the full-tendon transpositions may be considered. Another option in treating nonrestrictive DEP would be to match the duction deficit in the unaffected eye with a combined contralateral SR and IO recession.

Congenital Fibrosis of the Extraocular Muscles

CFEOM, usually autosomal dominant, is typically characterized by bilateral fibrosis of the IR with a secondary limitation of elevation and upper lid ptosis. Several variations in phenotype exist and may or may not be associated with other neurological or physical anomalies. Other extraocular muscles may be involved. Individuals affected with the classic type I CFEOM, described in our cases, usually assume a chin-up anomalous head posture. Surgical intervention can improve the ocular position and diminish the anomalous head posture. After intraoperative forced duction testing confirms the presence of a restricted IR, a large IR recession may be performed. An additional muscle hook retracting the tendon at its insertion may be required to safely place a suture within the restricted fibrotic muscle. Many smaller snips with scissors when disinserting the muscle can help prevent a scleral perforation. Simultaneous bilateral SO tenectomy may also assist in moving the eyes to primary gaze. In older children or adults with CFEOM who have binocularity, a posterior seventh or eighth SO tenectomy can be considered to preserve the anterior incyclotorsional fibers of the SO and thus prevent an intractable postoperative torsional diplopia.

Monocular CFEOM is very rare. Subtle abnormalities may be detected in the other eye. Case 12 has a monocular congenital fibrosis, which might also be classified as a restrictive monocular elevation deficiency due to IR restriction.

SUMMARY

Managing the strabismus syndromes discussed in this chapter can be humbling even for the most experienced strabismus surgeons. Nevertheless, with proper preoperative ocular motility measurements, interpretation of careful intraoperative forced duction testing, and familiarity with the surgical approaches outlined here, a patient with a complex strabismus syndrome can experience good ocular alignment, an expanded field of single binocular vision, and diminution of any preoperative anomalous head posture.

SUGGESTED READINGS

Bardorf CM, Baker JD. The efficacy of superior oblique split z tendon lengthening for superior oblique overaction. *J AAPOS*. 2003;7:96-102.

Snir M, Friling R, Kalish-Stiebel H, Bourla D, Weinberger D, Axer-Siegel R. Combined rectus muscle transposition with posterior fixation sutures for the treatment of double-elevator palsy. *Ophthalmology*. 2005;112(5):933-938.

Crawford JS. Late results of superior oblique muscle tenotomy in true Brown's syndrome. *Am J Ophthalmol*. 1980;89:824-829.

Crawford JS. Late results of superior oblique muscle tenotomy in true Brown's syndrome: incomitant strabismsus. *Am Orthopt J*. 1977;27:15-20.

Helveston EM. Surgical treatment of cyclic esotropia. *Am Orthopt J*. 1976;26:87-88.

Knapp P. The surgical treatment of double-elevator paralysis. *Trans Am Ophthalmol Soc*. 1969;67:304-323.

Kraft SP. A surgical approach for Duane syndrome. *J Pediatr Ophthalmol Strabismus*. 1988;25:119-129.

Kraft SP. Surgery for Duane syndrome. *Am Orthopt J*. 1993;43:18-26.

Kucak G, Kucak I. Selective management of double elevator palsy by either inferior rectus recession and/or Knapp type transposition surgery. *Binocul Vis Strabismus Q*. 1999;15:39-48.

Molarte AB, Rosenbaum AL. Vertical rectus muscle transposition surgery for Duane's syndrome. *J Pediatr Ophthalmol Strabismus*. 1990;27:171-177.

Rogers GL, Bremer DL. Surgical treatment of the upshoot and downshoot in Duane's retraction syndrome. *Ophthalmology*. 1984;91:1380-1383.

Rosenbaum AL. Costenbader lecture. The efficacy of rectus muscle transposition surgery in esotropic Duane syndrome and VI nerve palsy. *J AAPOS*. 2004;8:409-419.

Scott WE, Jackson OB. Double elevator palsy: the significance of the inferior rectus restriction. *Am Orthopt J*. 1977;27:5-10.

Sharma P, Saxena R, Rao BV, Menon V. Effect of posterior tenectomy of the superior oblique on objective and subjective torsion in cases of superior oblique overaction. *J Pediatr Ophthalmol Strabismus*. 2005;42(5):284-289.

Shin GS, Elliott RL, Rosenbaum AL. Posterior superior oblique tenectomy at the scleral insertion for collapse of A-pattern strabismus. *J Pediatr Ophthalmol Strabismus*. 1996;33(5):211-218.

Snir M, Friling R, Kalish-Stiebel H, et al. Strabismus surgery in children with Möbius syndrome. *J AAPOS*. 2000;4:58-59.

Stager DR, Parks MM, Stager DR, Pesheva M. Long-term results of silicone expander for moderate and severe Brown syndrome (Brown syndrome "plus"). *J AAPOS*. 1999;3:328-332.

Suh DW, Oystreck DT, Hunter DG. Long-term results of an intraoperative adjustable superior oblique tendon suture spacer using nonabsorbable suture for Brown syndrome. *Ophthalmology*. 2008;115:1800-1804.

Sun LL, Gole GA. Augmented vertical rectus (corrected) transposition for the treatment of strabismus in Möbius syndrome. *J AAPOS*. 2011;15(6):590-592.

Traboulsi EI, Jaafar MD, Kattan HM, Parks MM. Congenital fibrosis of the extraocular muscles: report of 24 cases illustrating the clinical spectrum of surgical management. *Am Orthopt J*. 1993;43:45-53.

Velez FG, Velez G, Thacker N. Superior oblique posterior tenectomy in patients with Brown syndrome with small deviations in the primary position. *J AAPOS*. 2006;10:214-219.

Waterhouse WJ, Enzenauer RW, Martyak AP. Successful strabismus surgery in a child with Möbius syndrome. *Ann Ophthalmol*. 1993;25:292-294.

Wright KW, Min BM, Park C. Comparison of superior oblique tendon expander to superior oblique tenotomy for the management of superior oblique overaction and Brown syndrome. *J Pediatr Ophthalmol Strabismus*. 1992;29:92-97.

Wright KW. Brown's syndrome: diagnosis and management. *Trans Am Ophthalmol Soc*. 1999;97:1023-1109.

Yang S, Mackinnon S, Dagi LR, Hunter DG. Superior rectus transposition vs medial rectus recession for treatment of esotropic Duane syndrome. *JAMA Ophthalmol*. 2014;132(6):669-675.

Yazdani A, Traboulsi EI. Classification and surgical management of patients with familial and sporadic forms of congenital fibrosis of the extraocular muscles. *Ophthalmology*. 2004;111(5):1035-1042.

Yurdakul NS, Ugurlu S, Maden A. Surgical treatment in patients with double elevator palsy. *Eur J Ophthalmol*. 2009;19(5):697-701.

7

Strabismus in Systemic Disease

Miles J. Burke, MD

Most physicians, including many ophthalmologists, consider strabismus an isolated disorder of eye muscle imbalance. Generally, they would be correct. However, pediatric ophthalmologists and adult strabismus specialists must always consider nonocular conditions that may be contributing to the ocular misalignment. These conditions include structural and developmental disorders of the skull and orbits (eg, craniosynostosis, Arnold-Chiari malformation, hydrocephalus), neuromuscular disease (eg, multiple sclerosis, myasthenia gravis, chronic progressive external ophthalmoplegia), metabolic disorders (eg, diabetes, thyroid disorders), infections (eg, orbital cellulitis, Gradenigo syndrome), and many other genetic and neoplastic conditions. Total care of these patients often requires working in consultation with other appropriate medical and surgical specialists. At the time of muscle surgery, the anesthetist must also be made aware of such disorders, which may increase the risk of anesthesia.

Case 1

A 60-year-old woman with thyroid orbitopathy has a 15-degree chin-up position to maintain both eyes in downgaze. She is unable to raise either eye even to the midline. Abduction and adduction are both slightly reduced.

Surgeon 1: Recess the BIR 5 mm on an adjustable suture.
Surgeon 2: Recess the BIR 5 mm.
Surgeon 3: Recess the BIR 9 mm.

Nelson LB, Levin AV, eds.
The Wills Eye Strabismus Surgery Handbook (pp 57-73).
© 2015 Taylor & Francis Group.

Case 2

A 40-year-old woman with thyroid disease has a right esotropia of 30 PD with a mild abduction deficit in the right eye.

Surgeon 1: Recess the BMR 5 mm OD adjustable.
Surgeon 2: Recess the RMR 7 mm. If this is a bilateral process, may need LMR recession too, but wait to determine effect of RMR recession.
Surgeon 3: Recess the RMR 7 mm.

Case 3

A 50-year-old man with thyroid disease has a 10-degree chin-up position, right hypotropia of 20 PD, and a mild elevation deficit of the right eye.

Surgeon 1: Recess the RIR 7 mm and the LIR 2.5 mm on adjustable sutures. Use additional 6-0 sutures to secure IRs if extremely tight.
Surgeon 2: Recess the RIR 6 mm.
Surgeon 3: Recess the RIR 7 mm.

Case 4

A 2-year-old boy with Apert syndrome has a right hypotropia of 20 PD and is unable to elevate the right eye past midline. Assume that horizontal recti and obliques are present and normally positioned.

Surgeon 1: Consider MRI of the orbits to determine if RSR is present or identify other abnormal muscles. Surgical plan depends on degree of restriction of RIR, presence of fusion on downgaze, and incomitancy of measurements in downgaze versus primary position. If significant restriction, recess the RIR. If absence of RSR or decreased function of RSR, then do a half-tendon-length upward transposition of the RMR and RLR. Recess the RIR if it is restricted. Do a full-tendon transfer to the RSR insertion area if the RIR is not restricted.
Surgeon 2: Image orbit to look for missing vertical muscles. If forced ductions are negative, perform Knapp procedure: RMR and RLR to RSR insertion area regardless of presence or absence of the RSR. If forced ductions are positive, recess the RIR.
Surgeon 3: Recess the RIR 7 mm, even if the RSR may be absent.

Case 5

A 5-year-old girl with complex craniosynostosis and a chin-up position. XT = 40 in primary position, which increases to XT = 60 in upgaze and decreases to 20 in downgaze. +4 elevation of adducting eye in side gaze.

Surgeon 1: Suspect rotation of the rectus muscles (MRI to confirm). Transpose a half tendon width both LR superiorly with 8-mm recession if LR significantly rotated alone (without IO recession). If LR OU not rotated, recess the LR OU 8 mm and recess the BIO 14 mm if overacting.

Surgeon 2: If the orbital bones have been stabilized by the craniofacial surgeon, consider imaging of the orbits to look for cyclorotation of muscles. Otherwise, recess the BLR 9 mm with displacement a half tendon width upward and also recess the BIO 14 mm without myectomy.

Surgeon 3: Recess the BLR 8 mm and anterior transposition of BIO temporal and parallel to the IR insertions.

Case 6

A 3-year-old girl with anterior plagiocephaly has a right head tilt of 10 degrees, left hypertropia of 12 PD in primary and left-gaze positions, left hypertropia of 16 PD in right gaze, +1 overaction of the left inferior oblique, and −3 underaction of the left superior oblique.

Surgeon 1: With a head tilt of only 10 degrees, SO tendon should be present. Do LSO tuck if the modified Guyton forced duction at time of surgery is grade 3 or 4. If it is grade 1 or 2, recess the LIO 14 mm.

Surgeon 2: Consider MRI of the extraocular muscles. If the LSO is absent, recess the LIO 4 mm posterior and just lateral to the LIR insertion without myectomy. If LSO is present, do LSO tuck.

Surgeon 3: Tuck the LSO.

Case 7

A 6-month-old child with Down syndrome has a 65-PD esotropia. There is only mild hyperopic refractive correction and no heart disease. Hyperopic spectacles did not improve the esotropia.

Surgeon 1: Try full hyperopic correction first, wait until age 12 months, then recess the BMR 6.5 mm adjustable.

Surgeon 2: Recess the BMR 6.5 mm.

Surgeon 3: Recess the BMR 6.5 mm.

Case 8

A 3-year-old with cerebral palsy has an alternating exotropia of 30 PD, minimal refractive error, and normal vision in each eye.

Surgeon 1: Wait until the child is 6 to 8 years old, then recess the BLR 6.5 mm adjustable.

Surgeon 2: If the XT measurements are stable over a 6-month period, recess the BLR 6 mm.

Surgeon 3: Recess 1 LR 9.5 mm.

Case 9

A 62-year-old with multiple sclerosis has bilateral internuclear ophthalmoplegia and an exotropia of 40 PD with diplopia.

Surgeon 1: Resect the BMR adjustable. Adjust postoperatively to 8- to 12-PD esotropia for distance considering expected postoperative drift.

Surgeon 2: Resect the BMR 6.5 mm.

Surgeon 3: Recess the BLR 8 mm.

Case 10

A 35-year-old on pyridostigmine for myasthenia gravis has a 3-year history of diplopia. The examination reveals 35 PD of right esotropia with a mild abduction deficit that has been stable for 1 year.

Surgeon 1: Recess the RMR 4 mm and the LMR 5.5 mm and place it on an adjustable suture. Goal is to leave patient esophoric. Warn patient that a second operation is likely within 2 to 5 years.

Surgeon 2: Recess the RMR 5 mm and resect the RLR 7 mm.

Surgeon 3: Recess the RMR 7 mm.

Case 11

A 10-year-old with Arnold-Chiari malformation has a comitant nonaccommodative esotropia of 30 PD.

Surgeon 1: If esotropia is recent, image posterior fossa and obtain neurosurgical consultation. If no neurosurgery is recommended, then recess the BMR 5.0 adjustable.

Surgeon 2: Consider neurosurgery for posterior fossa decompression because esotropia may resolve. If not, then recess the BMR 5 mm.

Surgeon 3: Recess the BMR 5 mm.

Case 12

A 73-year-old with Parkinson's disease has had double vision for 2 years with comitant esotropia of 15 PD.

Surgeon 1: First, try prisms. If prisms are not satisfactory, then recess the RMR or the LMR 5 mm adjustable.

Surgeon 2: Recess 1 MR 4.5 mm.

Surgeon 3: Recess 1 MR 4.5 mm

DISCUSSION

Cases 1, 2, and 3: Thyroid Orbitopathy

The first 3 cases involve strabismus associated with thyroid orbitopathy. These eye problems are caused by an autoimmune condition that produces factors that target fibroblasts, the support cells within the muscles, stimulating enlargement of the extraocular muscles. This enlargement causes the muscles to become inelastic, although normal contraction is typically preserved. Depending on the increased volume of the enlarged extraocular muscles, the globe may be pushed forward. This proptosis and the frequent retraction of the upper lids give the characteristic "stare" appearance. Orbital imaging, preferably MRI with contrast, can document which muscles are enlarged and provide information concerning possible optic nerve compression or stretch. Careful testing of visual acuity, visual field, pupil responses, and color saturation is helpful in evaluating optic nerve functions. When optic nerve concerns are present together with the concern of corneal exposure because of the magnitude of the proptosis, orbital decompression surgery may be necessary. Once the thyroid functions of a patient with thyroid orbitopathy have been normalized and the strabismic measurements are stable and reproducible over several months, one may entertain surgical realignment. Preoperative forced duction and forced generation testing help verify the functionality of the extraocular muscles. The inferior rectus muscle, followed by the medial rectus muscle, are the most frequently involved, although all of the extraocular muscles have been reported to be involved in thyroid orbitopathy. The primary surgical principle is to weaken the inelastic muscle or muscles to the point at which the eyes are aligned in primary position and, as much as one can obtain, in reading and downgaze positions. The use of adjustable sutures is preferred by many surgeons, given the unpredictable response of these abnormal muscles to surgery.

The surgeon must properly educate the patient that realignment in all gaze positions is often unobtainable and reoperations are common. Inelastic muscles will never be normal, residual areas of diplopia are common, and postoperative prisms and more eye muscle surgery are all very real possibilities. Patients with thyroid orbitopathy must also understand that orbital decompression and strabismus surgeries are completed before the upper eyelid retraction and the possible iatrogenic lower lid retraction (caused by large inferior rectus muscle recessions) are surgically managed.

Case 1 involves a patient with a 15-degree chin-up position associated with the inability to raise the eyes even to the midline. This represents a significant inelasticity of both inferior rectus muscles. Although no horizontal misalignment is measured, the extraocular movements suggest possible inelasticity of both the medial and lateral rectus muscles, or it may only be due to the significant inferior rectus inelasticity manifest in left- and right-gaze positions. An orbital scan would be very helpful in identifying which muscle or muscles are enlarged. The consultants and I are all in agreement on the need to recess both inferior rectus muscles. Two of the 3 respondents suggested measured recessions. One advised using adjustable sutures. Given most patients' small vertical fusional amplitudes, adjustability may have an advantage. Two of the 3 consultants wanted to recess 5 mm, whereas the third suggested 9-mm measured recessions. Larger recessions will yield more elevation but also risk underaction of downgaze, which may hamper ambulation, especially on stairs; it may also cause reading-position adjustment and make many other downgaze activities difficult, such as looking at one's plate while eating.

Case 2 involves a patient who has an abduction deficit of the right eye with a secondary 35-PD right esotropia. These findings suggest that there is more unilateral inelasticity of the right medial rectus muscle than of the left, although that should be checked carefully with preoperative forced duction testing. If one were to recess the right medial rectus muscle enough to eliminate the primary position 35 PD of esotropia, this amount of weakening would likely cause an exotropia for near fixation and an exotropia in the field of action of the right medial rectus muscle (left gaze). Two of the three consultants prefer a large 7-mm recession of the inelastic right medial rectus muscle. The third consultant advises a 5-mm bilateral recession of the medial rectus muscle while placing the tight right medial rectus muscle on an adjustable suture. A 7-mm unilateral recession may not straighten the eyes. Perhaps bilateral medial rectus recession with right medial rectus muscle adjustability has a higher chance of success, even though the right medial rectus muscle may have to be adjustably recessed more than 5 mm. Another option is asymmetric bilateral medial rectus muscle recessions, greater on the right (6 to 6.5 mm) than the left (5 mm). If one were completely sure that the left medial rectus had no evidence of thyroid orbitopathy, one could consider a recession of the right medial rectus muscle and a resection of the right lateral rectus muscle as a useful and safe alternative procedure.

In Case 3, a patient with thyroid orbitopathy is using a chin-up position to fuse in downgaze, presumably due to right inferior rectus muscle inelasticity. Computed tomography scans of the orbit and careful forced duction testing are recommended to assess the possibility of bilateral inferior rectus muscle involvement but with very asymmetric elevation deficits. One of the consultants was concerned enough about this potential to have advised bilateral asymmetric inferior rectus muscle recessions using an adjustable recession on the presumed less involved left inferior rectus muscle. The other 2 consultants recommend only a unilateral right inferior rectus muscle recession. With only 20 PD of hypotropia, a 6- or 7-mm inferior rectus muscle recession may overcorrect the hypotropia in downgaze and reading positions if not in primary position as well. If it could be determined that there was only right inferior rectus muscle involvement, one option would be to recess the right inferior rectus muscle only 4.5 mm; or, if involvement of the left inferior rectus cannot be excluded, recess the right inferior rectus muscle 6 mm and the left inferior rectus muscle 2 mm.

Cases 4, 5, and 6: Craniosynostoses

Craniosynostosis refers to premature closure of one or more of the cranial sutures, which results in abnormalities in the shape of the skull and/or orbit. Craniosynostosis may be isolated to one suture or present as multiple craniosynostoses, often part of a syndrome. Because of the associated abnormal orbital growth, optic atrophy is noted in up to 50% of some craniofacial disorders. The optic atrophy may be caused by chronic papilledema, narrowing of the optic canal, or kinking/stretching of the optic nerve due to the abnormal orbital shape. Strabismus and eye muscle abnormalities are particularly common manifestations of multiple craniosynostoses. Amblyopia is also common, typically due to astigmatism and anisometropia.

The molecular genetic basis of many of these syndromes has been elucidated, with several due to mutations in fibroblastic growth factor receptor genes. Like numerous other diseases once thought to be distinct entities, genetic analysis has demonstrated that these disorders are often variations along a spectrum of phenotypic expression for related genetic defects. The management of cranial and facial abnormalities of the craniosynostosis syndromes is surgical. The cranial vault is usually addressed first, followed by facial reconstruction. Strabismus is usually treated last.

Plagiocephaly is an isolated craniosynostosis that can involve either a coronal suture (anterior plagiocephaly) or a lambdoidal suture (posterior

plagiocephaly). The latter is not associated with strabismus. Posterior plagiocephaly may also occur in the absence of synostosis. These cases of
deformational posterior plagiocephaly are caused by a chronic prone
sleeping position or by in utero compressive forces. Unilateral coronal synostosis results in elevation of the brow and flattening of the forehead and
lateral orbital rim on the affected side. Frequent findings include ipsilateral
hypertropia and an abnormal head posture, usually a head tilt, which may
or may not be related to the strabismus. Nonocular torticollis is relatively
common and appears to be due to contraction or shortening of the ster-
nocleidomastoid muscle. This type of torticollis responds well to physical
therapy. Upward drifting of the ipsilateral adducting eye may mimic superi-
or oblique palsy or dissociated vertical deviation. This apparent underaction
of the superior oblique muscle results from the distortion of orbital anatomy
rather than a true fourth-nerve palsy.

Apert syndrome, also known as acrocephalosyndactyly, is an autosomal
dominant, multiple craniosynostoses syndrome associated with severe syn-
dactyly. Maxillary hypoplasia results in poor midfacial growth, leading to
retrusion of the lower forehead and shallow orbits, contributing to the typical exophthalmic appearance. Head shape can be variable but is most often
characterized by brachycephaly and turricephaly. Exophthalmos may be so
severe that the globe is actually positioned in front of the lids if not trapped
there. Other common manifestations include hypertelorism with lateral
splaying of the orbital walls, optic atrophy, exposure keratitis, amblyopia,
and strabismus. Eye muscle surgery is best performed after the skull and
facial reconstruction are complete.

In almost all of the craniosynostosis syndromes except saggital,
lambdoidal, and metopic isolated synostoses, the strabismologist must
be aware that unusual variations in extraocular anatomy may be present,
including missing muscles, duplicated muscles, anteriorly displaced muscle
insertions, muscularized intermuscular septum, bifid muscles, and muscles
placed to either side of the expected insertion sites. Excyclotorsion of the
globes may occur because of either an abnormal orbital configuration or
true anatomic malposition of the muscles. For example, the lateral rectus
muscle may be shifted downward, the medial rectus muscle upward, the
superior rectus muscle laterally, and the inferior rectus muscle medially.
These shifted muscles can cause the extraocular rotations to mimic inferior
oblique overaction and superior oblique underaction; this often causes a
V-pattern misalignment. Horizontal strabismus is found in 35% to 70% of
patients with craniosynostosis, with V-pattern exotropia being the most
common. Hypertropia of the adducting eye in side gaze can be dramatic
and mimic inferior oblique overaction even when no inferior oblique overaction is present. One of the surgical goals for the strabismus surgeon is

to determine what muscles are present and where they are located. This is very important in planning strabismus surgery. Coronal scans can be very helpful; MRI is preferable, but computed tomography gives excellent bony definition. At surgery, one must explore carefully to avoid inadvertently cutting a muscle that is not in the usual position. Limbal conjunctival incisions may be useful for this purpose.

In this case of Apert syndrome (Case 4) with poor elevation of the right eye and 20-PD hypotropia, all consultants appropriately requested more information. They all want scans to determine extraocular muscle positions and the presence or absence of the right superior rectus muscle. They all also want to know whether the right inferior rectus muscle is forced-duction tight. In the absence of a tight right inferior rectus muscle, 2 of the 3 advise full-tendon transposition of the right medial rectus and right lateral rectus muscles to the area of the right superior rectus muscle. If the right inferior rectus muscle were inelastic, all 3 would recess the right inferior rectus muscle. One of the 3 would also perform half-tendon transposition (ciliary artery sparing in the nontransposed half) of the right medial rectus and right lateral rectus muscles to the area of the right superior rectus muscle. One of the consultants also suggests a scenario in which the right superior rectus muscle is present and the hypotropia managed by a right inferior rectus muscle recession and left superior rectus muscle recession. I am in complete agreement with the consultants regarding the need to know the orbital and extraocular muscle configurations and the elasticity of the right inferior rectus before planning the surgical approach. I would follow the approach of full-tendon transpositions to the superior rectus if the inferior rectus muscle were not tight or a half-tendon transposition of both the medial and lateral rectus muscles to the right superior rectus and right inferior rectus recession if the right inferior rectus muscle were tight.

In Case 5, which involves a complex craniosynostosis with a large A pattern exotropia with significant, bilateral elevation in adduction, 2 of the 3 consultants specifically advised determining the presence of orbital excyclorotation. Two of the 3 consultants also advised elevating the lateral rectus muscles during the bilateral lateral rectus recession procedure, which was recommended by all the consultants. One of these 2 and the third consultant also advised either inferior oblique muscle recession or anterior transposition. In my opinion, the chin-up position, caused by the V pattern and the fusibility of a 20-PD intermittent exotropia, must be specifically addressed. I do not feel that partial-tendon-width supraplacement of the lateral rectus muscles alone will collapse a 40-PD difference from upgaze to downgaze. If coronal scans confirmed significant orbital excyclorotation, I would recess and superiorly transpose both lateral rectus muscles and also disinsert the medial rectus muscles and inferiorly transpose them, reattaching them on the circle of Tillaux. I would hold off on any inferior oblique surgery until the response to this first surgical procedure was determined.

Case 6 is that of a child with anterior plagiocephaly. One should use computed tomography scanning to evaluate the orbit and the extraocular muscle positions. Surgical treatment of this apparent left superior oblique palsy depends on the orbital configuration and the position and presence of the extraocular muscles. As long as the extraocular muscles are not abnormally rotated and this truly represents a right superior oblique muscle palsy, there will likely be torsional misalignment of the fundus. Since the examination suggests that there is more underaction of the superior oblique muscle than overaction of the inferior oblique muscle, a strengthening procedure on the superior oblique muscle should be considered. Two of the 3 consultants agree. The third consultant is concerned about the absence of the left superior oblique muscle and advises a left inferior oblique recession.

Case 7: Down Syndrome

Down syndrome, usually caused by complete trisomy of chromosome 21, is the most common chromosomal aberration in humans. Characteristic facial features, physical growth delay, and intellectual disability make Down syndrome easily distinguishable. Strabismus, usually esotropia, significant refractive errors, and amblyopia occur at a threefold increased incidence when compared with the general population. Refractive error, often high, is common. Patients may also have a multitude of other ocular abnormalities that should be considered in planning strabismus surgery and advising parents. These include nasolacrimal dysfunction, nystagmus, blepharitis, lid laxity, cataract, and optic nerve anomalies. These patients may also have systemic issues that can affect anesthesia, such as cervical spine instability and congenital heart disease. Although children with Down syndrome often present examination challenges, they usually respond well to the prescribed treatment plan. Therefore, when indicated, strabismus surgery should be performed to give such a child the best chance to develop binocular vision.

In Case 7, all 3 consultants concur with the normal responsiveness in children with Down syndrome to eye muscle surgery, using the standard recession amount for this 65-PD esotropia. One consultant suggested waiting until 12 months of age for a surgical correction. It was this consultant's suggestion that allowing more time for the child's developmental progress might improve the examiner's ability to obtain reliable measurements. This same consultant suggested using the adjustable recession technique. Data are needed regarding the utility of adjustable surgery specifically in patients with Down syndrome. Children with this condition may have an increased risk for anesthesia such that the surgeon should consider whether postoperative adjustments should be done under sedation or general anesthesia.

Case 8: Cerebral Palsy

Cerebral palsy is the general term for a group of permanent, nonprogressive movement disorders that cause physical disability and problems in development, mainly in areas of body movement. Most investigators believe that cerebral palsy is caused by damage to motor control centers in the developing brain, resulting in limitations of movement and postural instability. Impairments in cognition and epilepsy are common in patients with cerebral palsy. Assuming that there are developmental and cognitive delays, it may be challenging, on examination, to obtain reliable measurements. Therefore, reexamination may be necessary to ensure accuracy and stability. Most strabismologists recommend that the amount of eye muscle surgery not be altered in patients with cerebral palsy.

The consultants in Case 8 all consider these children to respond much as would a normal child, although some reduce their surgery by small amounts, such as 0.5 mm, with the thought that these muscles may be tighter, thus giving more effect per millimeter of surgery. I prefer a unilateral lateral rectus muscle recession and medial rectus muscle resection for a constant exotropia. In my experience, this improves convergence, helping to maintain the resulting surgical realignment. Others may find that bilateral lateral rectus muscle recession improves distance and near measurements equally; this is the procedure of choice for 2 of the 3 consultants. Single, large lateral rectus muscle recession procedures are often useful in patients with small-angle intermittent exotropia. However, in patients with constant exotropia, even a large lateral rectus recession is unlikely to afford a good realignment result. The last consultant prefers to wait until the child is several years older. Assuming that this child's examination findings are reliable at age 3 years, any delay should be balanced against the chances of early and better binocular function and normalizing this child's appearance. This will be helpful both for the child's self-image and for those who are already looking after the child because they would then see the child as less abnormal. These are good reasons not to delay surgery.

Case 9: Multiple Sclerosis

Multiple sclerosis is a disease that involves immune-related inflammatory attacks in which the insulating sheaths of nerve cells in the brain and spinal cord are damaged. This damaged myelin forms scar tissue (hence the name *sclerosis*) where the nerve fiber is damaged or destroyed. Thus, the nerve impulses traveling within and from the brain and spinal cord are distorted or disrupted, resulting in a wide range of signs and symptoms, both physical and mental. There is no cure for this disease, although promising new therapies are emerging. It typically presents between the ages of 20 and 50 years and has a 2-to-1 female-to-male predominance. Surgical plans should follow the usual numbers, but everyone must be aware of increased systemic risks of operation. Because this is a disorder that waxes and wanes, eye-movement disorders should be observed to ensure stable chronicity before proceeding with surgery. Optic neuritis can result in permanent visual loss in one or both eyes, further complicating the treatment plan.

The patient in Case 9, with large-angle exotropia and bilateral internuclear ophthalmoplegia, presents a very difficult management problem. Internuclear ophthalmoplegia is a disorder of conjugate lateral gaze in which the affected eye shows impairment of adduction. As a result, when the eyes attempt a lateral gaze, the eye on the affected side adducts only minimally. Convergence in these patients is generally preserved. In younger patients with bilateral internuclear ophthalmoplegia, multiple sclerosis is the most likely cause. In older patients, particularly with one-sided lesions, a stroke must be considered. Once the etiology is established and the misalignment stable, surgery may proceed.

The primary goal would be to align the eyes for primary position; if convergence is maintained, that should give the patient fusion in the central positions of gaze. Two of the 3 consultants suspect decreased convergence ability and underaction of the medial rectus muscles. To improve convergence, they advise resection of both medial rectus muscles. Both anticipate a slight postoperative drift outward, so their anticipated initial postoperative alignment would be a small-angle esotropia (10 to 12 PD). The third consultant anticipates normal convergence and advises a bilateral lateral rectus recession of the usual numbers for the measured exotropia angle. Given these surgical options, it is very important to determine the amplitudes of convergence in patients with bilateral internuclear ophthalmoplegia. Depending on this finding, I agree with the way in which the consultants would manage this case. As in all cases of functional problems of the extraocular muscles and incomitant deviations, the patient must be informed that fusion in both lateral gazes is difficult and unlikely to be achieved.

Case 10: Myasthenia Gravis

Myasthenia gravis is an autoimmune process resulting in damaged receptors on muscles or blockage of acetylcholine receptors at the postsynaptic neuromuscular junction by circulating antibodies. This results in a variable degree of muscle weakness that is often worse with fatigue or later in the day. Repeated attempts at moving or using a muscle result in a gradual increase in weakness of that muscle. Myasthenia gravis may affect swallowing and breathing, and both may represent serious health issues and anesthetic concerns. Myasthenia gravis is often associated with other autoimmune problems, such as thyroid orbitopathy. Proving the diagnosis of myasthenia gravis is often difficult and may, in some patients, be a diagnosis of exclusion. Blood tests such as acetylcholine receptor antibody and antimusk antibody testing are useful, but a significant percentage of patients have inconclusive or negative results. The sleep test is based on the characteristic of myasthenia gravis in which the symptoms and signs worsen with fatigue and improve after a period of rest. Myasthenia gravis can be confirmed by observing resolution of ptosis or diplopia immediately after a 30-minute period of sleep. The ice test consists of the application of an ice pack to the patient's symptomatic eye for 3 to 5 minutes. The response is positive when there is improvement of the diplopia or ptosis (decrease of at least 2 mm of the ptosis). Myasthenia gravis may respond when treated medically with acetylcholine esterase inhibitors or immunosuppressants (eg, steroids) and, in selected cases, thymectomy.

Myasthenia gravis may involve the levator palpebrae, causing ptosis, and/or weakened extraocular muscles, causing strabismus. If general body muscle weakness has not developed after 2 years of eye symptoms consistent with myasthenia gravis, it is generally considered that systemic involvement will not develop. Therefore, ocular myasthenia gravis should be considered a possible diagnosis in patients with the expected ocular findings but no systemic signs of myasthenia. In all cases of myasthenia gravis, spontaneous improvement with episodes of recurrence are typical, and the duration of muscle involvement is variable or may last for many years. Because most cases of strabismus in myasthenia gravis are due to muscle weakness, it can be challenging to balance the underaction and gaze deficits; however, doing so can maximize the patient's area of fusion. Care should be taken to avoid strabismus surgery unless the deviation is chronic and stable.

In Case 10, we have a 35-year-old patient taking pyridostigmine and having had double vision for 3 years. He had a stable abduction deficit for 1 year, leaving him with a primary position 35-PD esotropia, for which he requested surgical correction. In this patient, one would anticipate that the right esotropia was due to weakness of the right lateral rectus muscle. Since the diagnosis is not in doubt, no further workup of this patient would be necessary except for forced duction and forced generation testing in the office. My advice for surgical treatment in this case would be a right medial rectus recession and a right lateral rectus resection. This is in agreement with only 1 of the 3 consultants. Both of the others advise procedures attempting to balance the weakness of the right lateral rectus muscle. One suggests a large right medial rectus recession, anticipating that this would balance the horizontal muscles of the right eye and eliminate the esotropia by decreasing the adducting force against the weak right lateral rectus muscle. The other consultant would try to balance the forces using a small right medial rectus recession, helping to balance the right eye similarly as previously discussed, but also adding a larger weakening of the yoke of the weak right lateral rectus muscle by recessing the left medial rectus muscle. Therefore, by Hering's law, increased innervation will be necessary for the left medial rectus muscle to move into right gaze, and this increased innervation also goes to its yoke, hopefully improving right lateral muscle function.

Case 11: Arnold-Chiari Malformation

The Arnold-Chiari malformation consists of a downward displacement of the cerebellar tonsils through the foramen magnum, sometimes causing noncommunicating hydrocephalus due to the obstruction of cerebrospinal fluid outflow. There may be associated posterior fossa dysgenesis (Dandy-Walker malformation). Whenever Arnold-Chiari malformation is suspected or confirmed, neurosurgical consultation is mandatory. This condition is typically classified as being one of 4 types, with 1 being the most mild, asymptomatic, and usually benign. Types 3 and 4 are very rare. Type 2 is usually accompanied by a lumbar myelomeningocele, and there is often a larger cerebellar vermian displacement below the foramen magnum. The constellation of symptoms and signs of Arnold-Chiari malformation include scoliosis, headache, and neck pain with torticollis, often associated with variable oblique eye muscle dysfunction. This is the cause of the A- or V-pattern strabismus often associated with Arnold-Chiari malformation. Multiple cranial nerve palsies may also be seen. Strabismus surgery should not be entertained until secondary hydrocephalus is treated and the patient is stabilized by neurosurgery. It may be advisable to wait 6 months before strabismus repair to allow for any spontaneous improvement, as might be seen with other causes of new-onset cranial nerve palsies. Otherwise, the misalignments in Arnold-Chiari malformation respond well to typical surgical plans.

In Case 11, once neurosurgical consult has resolved the issue of the need for posterior fossa decompression, surgical treatment of the strabismus would be appropriate after enough time has passed to ensure that the deviation is quantitatively stable and any acquired cranial nerve palsy has been given the chance to recover function spontaneously (usually within 6 months). I agree with all 3 consultants, who advise bilateral medial rectus muscle recession.

Case 12: Parkinson's Disease

Parkinson's disease is a degenerative disorder of the central nervous system. Particular cells in the substantia nigra and the extrapyramidal system become impaired, resulting in the depletion of dopamine-secreting neurons. Dopamine is necessary for smooth and coordinated function of the body's muscles. The lack of dopamine causes the typical motor symptoms of Parkinsonism, including slowness of movement (bradykinesia), rigidity, tremor or involuntary shaking, and postural instability. These patients frequently have slow speech, often drool, and have an expressionless, almost masklike facial appearance. Nonmotor symptoms are common, including depression and anxiety, cognitive changes, and sleep disturbances. Ophthalmic involvement may cause impairment of voluntary horizontal and vertical gaze, resulting in jerkiness of the eye movements. It is fortunate that strabismus does not occur often in these patients, and, when surgery is necessary, good results using routine surgical numbers can be expected.

The patient in Case 12 has Parkinson's disease with a 15-PD esotropia, causing diplopia. Although one of the consultants suggests a trial of prisms before surgery, given that diplopia has been present for 2 years, nonsurgical remedies may already have been tried and have failed. All of the consultants advise one medial rectus recess; 2 would perform 4.5-mm recession and one a 5-mm adjustable recession. I am in agreement with these opinions. Medium-sized single medial rectus muscle recessions predictably correct 10 to 15 PD of misalignment. This would hopefully leave this patient with a small residual esophoria that could be controlled with fusion while nearly eliminating the possibility of an overcorrection.

SUGGESTED READINGS

Thyroid

Bothun ED, Scheurer RA, Harrison AR, Lee MS. Update on thyroid eye disease and management. *Binocul Vis Strabismus Q.* 2009;24(2):86-92.

Kim SH, Rotberg L, Sprunger DT. Standard strabismus surgery in thyroid ophthalmopathy. *Strabismus.* 2013;21(1):23-28.

Mainville NP, Jordan DR. Effect of orbital decompression on diplopia in thyroid-related orbitopathy. *Ophthalmol Plast Reconstr Surg.* 2014;30(2):137-140.

Nicholson BP, De Alba M, Perry JD, Traboulsi EI. Efficacy of the intraoperative relaxed muscle positioning technique in thyroid eye disease and analysis of cases requiring reoperation. *Clin Ophthalmol.* 2009;3:543-551.

Peragallo JH, Velez FG, Demer JL, Pineles SL. Postoperative drift in patients with thyroid ophthalmopathy undergoing unilateral inferior rectus muscle recession. *J AAPOS.* 2011;15(4):321-325.

Craniosynostosis

Dickman A, Parrilla R, Aliberti S, et al. Prevalence of neurological involvement and malformative/systemic syndromes in A- and V-pattern strabismus. *Ophthalm Epidemiol* 2012;19(5):302-305.

Forbes BJ, Pierce EA. Osseous and musculoskeletal disorders. In: Albert DM, Miller JW, Azar DT, Blodi BA, eds. *Albert and Jakobiec's Principles and Practice of Ophthalmology.* 3rd ed. Philadelphia, PA: Elsevier; 2008:

Guyton DL. Exaggerated traction test for the oblique muscles. *Ophthalmology.* 1981;88:1035-1040.

Holmes JM, Hatt SR, Leske DA. Superior oblique tucks for apparent inferior oblique overaction and V-pattern strabismus associated with craniosynostosis. *Strabismus.* 2010;18(3):111-115.

Matalia J, Kasturi N, Brodsky MC. Synostotic anterior plagiocephaly: a cause of familial congenital superior oblique muscle palsy. *Am Orthopt J.* 2013;63:80-84.

Rosenberg JB, Tepper OM, Medow NB. Strabismus in craniosynostosis. *J Pediatr Ophthalmol Strabismus.* 2013;50(3):140-148.

Down Syndrome

Motley WW III, Melson AT, Gray ME, Salisbury SR. Outcomes of strabismus surgery for esotropia in children with Down syndrome compared with matched controls. *J Pediatr Ophthalmol Strabismus.* 2012;49(4):211-214.

Stirn Kranjc B. Ocular abnormalities and systemic disease in Down syndrome. *Strabismus.* 2012;20(2):74-77.

Cerebral Palsy

Can CU, Polat S, Yasar M, Ilhan B, Altintas AG. Ocular alignment and results of strabismus surgery in neurologically impaired children. *Int J Ophthalmol.* 2012;5(1):113-115.

Fazzi E, Signorini SG, La Piana R, et al. Neuro-ophthalmological disorders in cerebral palsy: ophthalmological, oculomotor, and visual aspects. *Dev Med Child Neurol.* 2012;54(8):730-736.

Ma DJ, Yang HK, Hwang JM. Surgical outcomes of medial rectus recession in esotropia with cerebral palsy. *Ophthalmology.* 2013;120(4):663-667.

Multiple Sclerosis

Adams WE, Leavitt JA, Holmes JM. Strabismus surgery for internuclear ophthalmoplegia with exotropia in multiple sclerosis. *J AAPOS.* 2009;13(1):13-15.

Jenkins PF. The multiple facets of multiple sclerosis. *Am Orthopt J.* 2007;57:69-78.

Myasthenia Gravis

Cleary M, Williams GJ, Metcalfe RA. The pattern of extra-ocular muscle involvement in ocular myasthenia. *Strabismus.* 2008;16(1):11-18.

Haines SR, Thurtell MJ. Treatment of ocular myasthenia gravis. *Curr Treat Options Neurol.* 2012;14(1):103-112.

Kushner BJ, ed. Grand rounds #16: a case of myasthenia gravis with extraocular pareses. *Binocul Vision Q.* 1989;4(4):187-192.

Peragallo JH, Velez FG, Demer JL, Pineles SL. Long-term follow-up of strabismus surgery for patients with ocular myasthenia gravis. *J Neuro-ophthalmol.* 2013;33(1):40-44.

Arnold-Chiari Malformation

Kowal L, Yahalom C, Shuey NH. Chiari 1 malformation presenting as strabismus. *Binocul Vis Strabismus Q.* 2006;21(1):18-26.

Rech L, Mehta V, MacDonald IM. Esotropia and Chiari 1 malformation: report of a case and review of outcomes of posterior fossa decompression and strabismus surgery. *Can J Ophthalmol.* 2013;48(4):e90-e92.

Parkinson's Disease

Repka MX, Claro MC, Loupe DN, Reich SG. Ocular motility in Parkinson's disease. *J Pediatr Ophthalmol Strabismus.* 1996;33(3):144-147.

8

Other Complex Strabismus Cases

Kammi Gunton, MD

In approaching complex strabismus cases, the goals of strabismus surgery may vary from those of routine cases. The goal of surgery for complex cases may be the elimination of diplopia in the primary position, reestablishment of bifixation, restoration of some binocularity, reduction of incomitance to allow prismatic correction, restoration of socially acceptable alignment, or some combination of the above. The potential for bifixation and/or binocularity must be conscientiously addressed. In some cases, both bifixation and binocularity are possible, whereas binocularity alone may be the goal for patients with poor visual acuity or central scotoma. Preoperative sensory examination can be insightful regarding the potential for binocularity, but it is not always conclusive. In all cases, the expected outcome must be discussed with the patient so that the patient's and surgeon's goals are completely understood and aligned.

In adult patients with prior bifixation and good visual acuity in each eye, trauma, ophthalmic surgery, or otolaryngologic surgery can result in restrictive strabismus due to scarring of an extraocular muscle with resulting incomitance. In these cases, the primary goal of strabismus surgery may be the restoration of bifixation in the primary position alone. Secondarily, surgery may be tailored to reduce the incomitance. Discussions with retina and glaucoma specialists regarding removal of any restricting devices/apparatus should occur before the surgical procedures. In some

Nelson LB, Levin AV, eds.
The Wills Eye Strabismus Surgery Handbook (pp 75-86).

cases, collaboration in the operating room can assist in providing the best care. Although incomitance creates significant symptoms, eliminating all incomitance is not always achievable. Clear communication with patients regarding the possibility of persistent incomitance is vital.

In other cases, there is limited potential for bifixation, as in the setting of poor visual acuity. In addition, adults without suppression scotomas may have a very narrow window of alignment that relieves diplopia. Prisms may be needed after surgery. Adults with suppression scotomas from childhood or scotomas from retinal disease may require a final alignment that differs from orthotropia to achieve comfortable vision. In the latter setting, a trial of prismatic correction either in the office or as a Fresnel applique to glasses can often help to predict whether symptomatic improvement will occur.

Finally, the goal of restoring socially acceptable alignment cannot be minimized. Strabismus surgery should be proposed to maintain acceptable alignment as long as possible. Consecutive exotropia following nonaccommodative esotropia can occur, and patients with persistent hyperopia must be prepared for recurrent accommodative esotropia in the absence of binocular function. Multiple previous strabismus surgeries also influence surgical plans.

A clear delineation of the goals of surgery—whether bifixation, binocularity, relief of diplopia in the primary position, or socially acceptable alignment—must be discussed and mutually agreed upon by the surgeon and the patient to achieve a satisfactory outcome.

Case 1

A 9-year-old aphake OD with microphthalmia following persistent fetal vasculature wearing contact lens. Vision OD 20/60. No longer patching for ambylopia.

a. RET = 30, corneal diameter = 7.5.

Surgeon 1: Recess the RMR 6 mm on adjustable suture. Adjust to esophoria of 6 to 8 PD.

Surgeon 2: Recess the RMR 6 mm.

Surgeon 3: Recess the RMR 3.5 mm and resect the RLR 4 mm.

b. RET = 45, corneal diameter = 7.5.

Surgeon 1: Recess the RMR 5 mm and resect the RLR 6 mm on adjustable suture.

Surgeon 2: If eye is smaller by A-scan, recess the RMR 5 mm and resect the RLR 7 mm.

Surgeon 3: Recess the RMR 4 mm and resect the RLR 5 mm.

c. ET = 45, corneal diameter = 10.

   Surgeon 1: Recess the BMR 5.5 mm adjustable.

   Surgeon 2: Recess the RMR 5.5 mm and resect the RLR 8 mm.

   Surgeon 3: Recess the RMR 5 mm and resect the RLR 6 mm.

Case 2

Aphakia OU in contact lenses, equal vision, no nystagmus, corneal diameter 7, AET = 50.

   Surgeon 1: Recess the BMR 5.5 mm both on adjustable.

   Surgeon 2: Recess the BMR 5.5 mm.

   Surgeon 3: Recess the BMR 4 mm.

Case 3

A 30-year-old with scleral buckle OD, vision with glasses OD 20/80, OS 20/20, diplopia.

a. RXT = 20.

   Surgeon 1: Possibly remove scleral buckle (consult with retinal surgeon; usually easy to do but not necessary in all cases). Do forced ductions if there is restriction to adduction on forced duction tests, then recess the RLR until the eye can be adducted almost fully. Start with RLR recession of 8 mm. If the eye still cannot be adducted easily, recess the RLR more until adduction becomes almost full. The eye should appear straight on the table. If the eye still appears XT despite recessing the RLR 13 mm, then add resection or plication of the MR.

   Surgeon 2: Recess the RLR 8 mm.

   Surgeon 3: Recess the RLR 4 mm and resect the RMR 3 mm. Hang back sutures depending on buckle location.

b. V pattern RET = 20 in primary position, 15 upgaze, 35 downgaze.

   Surgeon 1: Remove buckle around the RMR and recess the RMR 5.5 mm adjustable. If the RMR is too superior, infraplace one-half tendon width or more depending on location at time of surgery.

   Surgeon 2: Recess the RMR 5.5 mm and ignore V pattern.

   Surgeon 3: Resect the RLR 4 mm and recess the RMR 3.5 mm with three-quarters-tendon-width downshift.

Case 4

Adult with superior temporal trabeculectomy OS performed with mitomycin, vision OS 20/100, OD 20/20 with no glaucoma 20/20.

a. LXT = 20.

Surgeon 1: Plicate or resect the LMR 5 mm adjustable.

Surgeon 2: Resect the LMR 6 mm. Warn patient of risk of trabeculectomy failure and discuss option for surgery OD.

Surgeon 3: Recess the LLR 4 mm and resect the LMR 3 mm using inferior fornix approach.

b. LXT = 50.

Surgeon 1: Recess the RLR 9 mm nonadjustable after thorough discussion with family regarding risk/benefit of operating on good eye; resect/plicate the LMR 5 mm adjustable.

Surgeon 2: Recess the RLR 9 mm and resect the RMR 6 mm.

Surgeon 3: Recess the LLR 8 mm and resect the LMR 6 mm using inferior fornix approach.

Case 5

A 35-year-old with accommodative esotropia had LASIK surgery for his hyperopia. Complaining of diplopia. AET = 35.

Surgeon 1: Make sure no residual hyperopia by cycloplegic refraction. Recess the BMR 5 mm adjustable.

Surgeon 2: Recess the BMR 5 mm.

Surgeon 3: Assess for residual hyperopia; if present, enhance LASIK, then reassess. If emmetropic, recess the MR 4 mm and resect the LR 5 mm of dominant eye.

Case 6

Traumatic transection of the RIR 6 mm posterior to the insertion, globe intact. Preoperative RHT = 30 with complete depression deficit.

Surgeon 1: First, determine whether the RIR muscle can be found. MRI scan may be helpful. If found, then suture the torn piece of the RIR to the remaining intact RIR muscle. If transected RIR cannot be found, then a half-tendon transposition of RMR and RLR to either side of the insertion of the RIR. Lateral fixation (Foster) sutures placed 6 mm from insertion with 6-0 nonabsorbable suture (on either side of the

RIR). Recess the LIR muscle if RHT still present on the table; recess until eyes appear straight. LIR muscle is placed on adjustable suture and adjusted until eyes appear in primary position on the table.

Surgeon 2: Explore and try to repair right inferior rectus. If right inferior rectus not found, anteriorize right inferior oblique 1 to 2 mm anterior to temporal border of the RIR insertion.

Surgeon 3: Explain to the patient that this may be a staged procedure. Explore RIR for possible reattachment. If proximal end found, reattach and reassess in clinic. If unable to find, then Knapp procedure with full-tendon-width transposition of the RMR and RLR to the insertion of the RIR in the spiral of Tillaux. If anterior segment ischemia is a concern, consider inferior half of each horizontal rectus for transposition.

Case 7

After recurrent medial pterygium excision OD, RXT = 35 with inability to adduct OD past the midline and diplopia.

Surgeon 1: RMR needs to be advanced/plicated or resected a total of 4 mm. For example, if the RMR is found 8 mm from the limbus, it should be advanced to 5.5 from the limbus and resected 1.5 mm on an adjustable suture. If the RMR is lost, then determine whether the RLR is tight by forced duction tests. Recess the RLR on an adjustable suture until eye can be adducted almost completely. Then, perform half-tendon transposition of the RIR and RSR to either side of the original insertion (5.5 from the limbus) of the RMR. If the forced duction tests are normal, the RLR muscle need not be recessed, but augment the half-tendon transposition of the RIR and RSR by placing a Foster suture with a 6-0 nonabsorbable suture 8 mm from the insertion of the RMR (13.5 mm from the limbus).

Surgeon 2: Suspect lost right medial rectus. Explore and repair right medial rectus. If medial rectus not found, transpose the nasal half of the RSR and RIR to the insertion of lost medial rectus.

Surgeon 3: Must explain to patient that this may be a staged procedure. Explore RMR for possible reattachment. If proximal end found, reattach and reassess in clinic. If unable to find, then full tendon transposition of the RSR and RIR to the old insertion of the RMR in the Spiral of Tillaux. If anterior segment ischemia is a concern, then consider transposing only medial half of each horizontal rectus.

Case 8

After a glaucoma tube at the 2-o'clock position OD, vertical diplopia noted. VA OD 20/100, OS 20/30. Mild depression deficit. Diplopia has persisted for 6 months. RHT = 15.

Surgeon 1: Plicate or resect the RIR 4 mm adjustable.

Surgeon 2: Recess the RSR 6 mm. May have a fibrous capsule from tube plate restricting eye movement that may need to be removed. Would have a glaucoma surgeon involved with the strabismus surgery because the tube will likely need to be revised.

Surgeon 3: Patient likely does not want OS touched, so would consider resecting the RIR 5 mm. Consider adjustable.

Case 9

"Morning glory" syndrome OD in a 7-year-old boy. VA OD 20/200, OS 20/25. RET = 45, RHT = 15.

Surgeon 1: Recess the RMR 5 mm adjustable with half-or-more-tendon-width transposition inferiorly; resect the RLR 8 mm adjustable with half-tendon-width transposition inferiorly.

Surgeon 2: Recess the RMR 5.5 mm and resect the RLR 8 mm. Transpose both recti one-half tendon width down.

Surgeon 3: Recess the RMR 5 mm and resect the RLR 6 mm, each with full-tendon-width downshift.

Case 10

Third corneal transplant OD, stable for 1 year. VA OD 20/50, OS 20/20. RXT = 40.

Surgeon 1: Resect the LMR 6 mm and recess the LLR 8 mm.

Surgeon 2: Recess the RLR 8 mm and resect the RMR 5 mm. Would warn of risk of graft failure and discuss option of procedure on OS.

Surgeon 3: Resect the RMR 6 mm and recess the RLR 8 mm. Fornix approach avoiding limbal vessels. Consider extra steroid drops post-operatively.

Case 11

A 60-year-old with a history of amblyopia OD. Has cataract surgery OD, now VA OD 20/50, OS 20/30. Noted onset of diplopia after cataract surgery. RXT = 25.

Surgeon 1: Recess the RLR 6.5 mm adjustable and resect the RMR 4.0 mm adjustable.

Surgeon 2: Recess the RLR 9 mm.

Surgeon 3: Resect the RMR 4 mm and recess the RLR 6 mm.

DISCUSSION

In approaching each of these cases, assessment of the potential for binocularity is the first consideration. Binocularity is influenced by early visual experience, amblyopia, poor visual acuity, and the presence or absence of suppression scotomas. Sensory test results provide an estimation of the potential for binocularity.[1-3] Worth 4-dot and red lens testing should be attempted with prismatic correction provided to achieve orthotropia. If the patient reports fusion with Worth 4-dot and prismatic correction, binocularity can be expected postoperatively. Differences in the responses to near and distance targets in Worth 4-dot testing reveal the size of any suppression scotomas. In adult patients, subjective responses can be employed to further refine the misalignment or relieve diplopia/visual discomfort. Fusion with the red lens on a specific target reveals the potential for bifixation and estimates fusional vergences. Many patients have fusional amplitudes that can be measured to give a range of acceptable alignment to relieve their symptoms. The red lens can also reveal the extent of suppression scotomas. If patients report continued diplopia with prismatic correction preoperatively, there is a greater possibility of diplopia following surgery, although Kushner found that of the patients reporting diplopia with prismatic correction choosing to proceed with surgery, only 2% had persistent diplopia postoperatively.[3] Sensory testing data are invaluable in planning strabismus procedures.

Many cases involve patients with reduced binocular function, such as the cases of persistent fetal vasculature with reduced visual acuity, morning glory syndrome, unilateral aphakia, and amblyopia. In these circumstances, bifixation cannot be achieved. Binocularity may be possible, but often, socially acceptable alignment is the goal. Factors that influence the desired alignment include the interpupillary distance, the width of the patient's face, corneal diameters, axial length, the patient's age, and the likely progression of the alignment postoperatively. Facial biometry's influence on strabismus surgery has not been well studied. When the goal is socially acceptable alignment, placing the prismatic correction in front of the dominant eye and observing the position of the nondominant eye allows the patient via a mirror and/or accompanying family members to assess the change in alignment expected from the surgery for a particular prismatic correction. Often, the desired alignment can differ from the measured misalignment due to facial features. In addition, when patients are wearing their refractive correction, large refractive errors influence the measured misalignment. The deviation is changed by 2.5% per diopter of spherical refraction. Myopic refraction causes measurements greater than the true deviation and hyperopic refraction causes less. Shorter axial lengths with large hyperopic corrections must be taken into consideration in determining surgical dosage.

The tables used to calculate the amount of surgery on rectus muscles are based on previous surgical experience. The numbers are generally not revised on the basis of a patient's age except in very large recessions, despite the shorter axial length in children. Although Kushner found that a patient's age, axial length, and refractive error influenced the location of the medial rectus muscle from the limbus and found a statistically significant inverse correlation between axial length and the number of millimeters of recession required of the medial rectus, these factors ultimately did not significantly influence the clinical response to strabismus surgery in children.[4,5] Ultrasound biomicroscopy can be employed in unusual cases to determine the preoperative location of the insertion of a rectus muscle, but it is generally not required.[6] In microphthalmia, the relationship between the insertion and the equator would differ significantly from that in normal-sized eyes. Large recessions over 2 mm posterior to the equator of the eye might result in a limitation in gaze and underaction of the involved muscle.[7] An eye with persistent fetal vasculature would be expected to have a significantly shorter axial length. Small corneal diameters would also be expected as a manifestation of microphthalmia. Therefore, very large recessions of the medial rectus may place the muscle posterior to the equator to an extent that causes a limitation in adduction. Conservative recessions of the medial rectus in this setting address both this concern and the high potential for consecutive exotropia over time due to lack of binocularity. Adult patients become more exotropic with the gradual reduction in their hyperopic correction with age. Taking the 2 factors of smaller corneas and poor binocular potential into account, surgery for esotropia in the setting of amblyopia or reduced visual acuity in one eye may aim for some undercorrection of the deviation.

In another group of cases, restrictive strabismus is present. Strabismus requiring prism or surgical correction has been reported in as many as 23% of cases following scleral buckle.[8] The patterns of strabismus vary widely, with some limitations in ductions present in 73% of patients. Restriction of motility may indicate mechanical obstruction created by the buckle and is more common with encircling scleral buckles. In addition, extraocular muscles can be disinserted at the buckle, sometimes owing to anterior migration of the silicone element with transection of the muscle seen on MRI.[9] Torsion also occurs either because of induced superior oblique palsy or tightening of the inferior rectus from the buckle.[10] In patients with strabismus secondary to scleral buckles, the success rates of strabismus surgery with correction of a deviation to within 10 PD of orthotropia vary between 33% and 72%.[11,12] Success was associated with smaller preoperative deviations. Removal of the scleral buckle did not influence the success rate in one study[12] but increased the success rate from 10% to 62% in another.[11] The use of adjustable sutures tended to improve success but did not reach statistical significance.[11] Many surgeons who detect restrictions preoperatively will consult with retinal specialists regarding removal of the buckle to improve the motility, considering also the risk for retinal redetachment. Forced ductions should be performed prior to surgery, as they can help to guide the surgical plan. When the buckle is not removed, hooking the muscle can present technical difficulties, especially when incisions are made over scarred conjunctiva. Reattaching the muscle is simpler with large recessions posterior to the buckle or if a hang-back technique is utilized. The goal of surgery should be resolution of diplopia in the primary position. Finally, it should be mentioned that many cases of strabismus after retinal detachment are the result of sensory strabismus without surgical restriction.

Glaucoma drainage tube shunts and high blebs can also result in restrictive strabismus. Studies have found the risk for developing diplopia following tube placement to be 1.4% in adults.[13] In children, the rate of strabismus was much higher, at 57% in congenital glaucoma.[14] The mean time to onset of diplopia following glaucoma drainage surgery was 2 months.[13] The larger the implant, the greater the chance of developing diplopia. In some patients, diplopia immediately following glaucoma surgery may resolve spontaneously within 6 months. With persistent diplopia, scarring of the muscle within the bleb, splitting of the muscle by the plate, or impingement of the muscle by the edge of the implant must be considered. In one study following patients with double-plate Molteno implantation, 46% of the patients developed a motility disturbance.[15] In this study, the etiology of the strabismus was restriction of the superior rectus and superior oblique (1 of 3), acquired Brown syndrome (1 of 3), superior oblique palsy (1 of 3), and one case of lateral rectus palsy.[15] Forced ductions can be helpful in determining the etiology. In addition, preservation of a functional bleb should be considered in the plan for strabismus surgery. Preoperative discussion of complications should include failure of the bleb and the need for additional glaucoma surgery. Conjunctival cul-de-sac incisions away from the bleb would be given priority. Unless there is obvious restriction, surgery on the muscle adjacent to the bleb should be avoided.

Corneal transplants present a different consideration in regard to strabismus surgery. Corneal graft failure secondary to problems with the external surface of the graft is as common as failure due to immunological rejection.[16] Strabismus surgery has not been reported to predispose to graft failure, but it does influence the external ocular surface. Goblet cell depletion following strabismus surgery results in tear film instability. In one study, tear-film composition did not return to baseline levels until 4 months after strabismus surgery.[17] Immediately after strabismus surgery, increased lubrication of the ocular surface and increased monitoring by corneal specialists may diminish the risk of graft failure. The risk of corneal graft rejection should be addressed with patients with strabismus preoperatively.

One of the most difficult strabismus cases involves a slipped or lost muscle. Rectus muscles may be lost due to direct trauma, sinus surgery, or ophthalmic surgery. The first priority should be given to retrieving the muscle. Forced ductions, active force generation, and orbital imaging studies can help diagnose a lost muscle. Techniques for retrieval include searching in Tenon's layer in the quadrant of the slipped muscle, transcutaneous medial orbitotomy, or endoscopy.[18] Imaging studies, including MRI with surface coils and computed tomography with an image guidance system, may also be useful. Experience with these systems is limited to a few published cases.[19,20] If the muscle cannot be retrieved, transpositions must be considered to restore tone and improve the alignment in primary position. Alignment in the primary position is prioritized over the restoration of ductions.

There are many different transposition procedures. Full-tendon transpositions of the 2 adjacent rectus muscles in a Knapp transposition are placed along the spiral of Tillaux next to the weak/paralyzed muscle. In a Hummelsheim procedure, the transposed muscles are split in half, and only the halves adjacent to the paralyzed muscle are transposed. Another surgery that preserves the ciliary arteries is the Jensen procedure, which splits both the transposed muscles and the weak muscle along their long axis. Then, without disinsertion, the corresponding halves are tied together with nonabsorbable suture. Recently, a lateral fixation suture augmentation or Foster suture further enhanced the effect of a full-tendon transposition. A nonabsorbable suture is placed through approximately one-quarter of the muscle width, 8 mm from the insertion of the transposed muscle, and passed 8 mm posterior to the insertion of the weak muscle.[21] Transposition of the superior rectus muscle alone instead of both the superior and inferior rectus muscles to the adjacent palsied lateral rectus has been shown to be an effective transposition without significant complications of postoperative vertical tropias.[22]

Refractive procedures are increasingly common and present a different challenge to the strabismus surgeon. LASIK or LASEK to treat hyperopia and fully accommodative esotropia in adults has been studied.[23-26] Over time, regression with recurrence of hyperopia and accommodative strabismus have been shown to occur. At 2-year follow-up after LASEK, 78% of patients maintained refraction within ±0.50 D of intended correction.[24] With residual hyperopia postoperatively or regression of correction, accommodative esotropia may also recur. The first line of treatment would be rerefraction and correction of any hyperopia. If the deviation resolves with hyperopic correction, retreatment with LASIK or other refractive options should be considered and discussed with the refractive surgeon. If the deviation is not responsive to refractive correction, surgical options or prismatic correction as in cases of nonaccommodative esotropia should be employed.

As the cases presented here show, strabismus surgery can be challenging but also highly rewarding. With the consideration of binocular potential, socially acceptable alignment, elimination of diplopia, and reduction in incomitance, goals must be carefully addressed with patients. Realistic expectations can help to prevent patient dissatisfaction.

REFERENCES

1. Morrison D, McSwain W, Donahue S. Comparison of sensory outcomes in patients with monofixation versus bifoveal fusion after surgery for intermittent exotropia. *J AAPOS.* 2010;14:47-51.
2. Dickmann A, Aliberti S, Rebecchi MT, et al. Improved sensory status and quality-of-life measures in adult patients after strabismus surgery. *J AAPOS* 2013;17:25-28.
3. Kushner BJ. Intractable diplopia after strabismus surgery in adults. *Arch Ophthalmol.* 2002;120:1498-1504.
4. Kushner BJ, Lucchese NJ, Morton GV. The influence of axial length on the response to strabismus surgery. *Arch Ophthalmol.* 1989;107:1616-1618.
5. Kushner BJ, Fisher MR, Lucchese NJ, Morton GV. Factors influencing response to strabismus surgery. *Arch Ophthalmol.* 1993;111:75-79.
6. Watts P, Smith D, Mackeen L, et al. Evaluation of the ultrasound biomicroscopy in strabismus surgery. *J AAPOS.* 2002;6:187-190.
7. Kushner BJ, Fisher MR, Lucchese NJ, Morton GV. How far can a medial rectus safely be recessed? *J Pediatr Ophthalmol Strabismus.* 1994;31:138-146.
8. Smiddy WE, Loupe D, Michels RG, et al. Extraocular muscle imbalance after scleral buckling surgery. *Ophthalmology.* 1989;96:1485-1489.
9. Wu TE, Rosenbaum AL, Demer JL. Severe strabismus after scleral buckling: multiple mechanisms revealed by high-resolution magnetic resonance imaging. *Ophthalmology.* 2005;112:327-336.
10. Cooper LL, Harrison S, Rosenbaum AL. Ocular torsion as a complication of scleral buckle procedures for retinal detachments. *J AAPOS.* 1998;2:279-284.
11. Chang JH, Hutchinson AK, Zhang M, et al. Strabismus surgery outcomes after scleral buckling procedures for retinal reattachment. *Strabismus.* 2013;21:235-241.
12. Rabinowitz R, Velez RG, Pineles SL. Risk factors influencing the outcome of strabismus surgery following retinal detachment surgery with scleral buckle. *J AAPOS.* 2013;17:594-597.

13. Abdelaziz A, Capo H, Banitt MR, et al. Diplopia after glaucoma drainage device implantation. *J AAPOS*. 2013;17:192-196.
14. O'Malley Schotthoefer E, Yanovitch TL, Freedman SF. Aqueous drainage device surgery in refractory pediatric glaucoma: II. Ocular motility consequences. *J AAPOS*. 2008;12:40-45.
15. Dobler-Dixon AA, Cantor LB, Sondhi N, et al. Prospective evaluation of extraocular motility following double-plate Molteno implantation. *Arch Ophthalmol*. 1999;117:1155-1160.
16. Price FW, Whitson WE, Collins KS, Marks RG. Five-year corneal graft survival. A large, single-center patient cohort. *Arch Ophthalmol*. 1993;111:799-805.
17. Jeon S, Park SH, Choi JS, Shin SY. Ocular surface changes after lateral rectus recession. *Ophthalmic Surg Lasers Imaging*. 2011;42:428-433.
18. Lenart TD, Reichman OS, McMahon SJ, et al. Retrieval of lost medial rectus muscles with a combined ophthalmologic and otolaryngologic surgical approach. *Am J Ophthalmol*. 2000;130:645-652.
19. Srivastava SK, Reichman OS, Lambert SR. The use of an image guidance system in retrieving lost medial rectus muscles. *J AAPOS*. 2002;6:309-314.
20. Pineles SL, Laursen J, Goldberg RA, et al. Function of transected or avulsed rectus muscles following recovery using an anterior orbitotomy approach. *J AAPOS*. 2012;16:336-341.
21. Foster RS. Vertical muscle transposition augmented with lateral fixation. *J AAPOS*. 1997;1:20-30.
22. Mehendale RA, Dagi LR, Wu C, et al. Superior rectus transposition and medial rectus recession for Duane syndrome and sixth nerve palsy. *Arch Ophthalmol*. 2012;130:195-201.
23. Brugnoli de Pagano OM, Pagano GL. Laser in situ keratomileusis for the treatment of refractive accommodative esotropia. *Ophthalmology*. 2012;119:159-163.
24. Autrata R, Rehurek J. Laser-assisted subepithelial keractectomy and photorefractive keractectomy in the correction of hyperopia. *J Cataract Refract Surg*. 2003;29:2105-2114.
25. Kirwan C, O'Keefe M, O'Mullane GM, Sheehan C. Refractive surgery in patients with accommodative and non-accommodative strabismus: 1-year prospective follow-up. *Br J Ophthalmol*. 2010;94:898-902.
26. Settas G, Settas C, Minos E, Yeung IY. Photorefractive keratectomy (PRK) versus laser assisted in situ keratomileusis for hyperopic correction. *Cochrane Database Syst Rev*. 2012;(6):CD007112.

9

Reoperations

Rudolph S. Wagner, MD

The ability to achieve good results with strabismus surgery reoperations depends on many factors, not the least of which is careful preoperative planning. Unexpected intraoperative findings—including extensive scar tissue formation, anomalous muscle insertion or location, or a slipped muscle—can occur, and the surgeon must be ready to make rapid yet well-thought-out decisions. Many surgeons follow Cooper's law, which suggests that undoing what was done is not always the best way to overcome an overcorrection.[1] Rather, the surgical decision should be based on the result of the examination and not the fact that the patient had prior surgery. This dictum may not always apply—for example, in cases of a slipped muscle that must be advanced—but it remains generally good advice. It is technically easier to operate on muscles that have not undergone prior surgery, but in many cases, restrictive forces must be relieved by reoperation of the involved muscle.

History of previous surgery should be obtained but is not always detailed or accurate. Operative reports from the previous surgeries are helpful. Keep in mind that surgeons may use different reference points for their graded measurements (eg, posterior versus anterior insertion). At the very least, it is useful to know whether the original strabismus was an esotropia or exotropia and if there was a vertical component. Ask if surgery was performed on one or both eyes. Most patients will remember if an adjustable

Nelson LB, Levin AV, eds.
The Wills Eye Strabismus Surgery Handbook (pp 87-97).
© 2015 Taylor & Francis Group.

suture was used or if some untoward event occurred in the perioperative period. A variety of imaging techniques have been reported to be useful in determining the location of the muscle in cases of a suspected "lost" muscle.[2,3]

As generally used in planning any strabismus surgery, best corrected visual acuity, fixation preference, and the potential for binocular vision should be assessed. Careful measurements in all fields of gaze at distance and near fixation should be performed. Slit-lamp examination is useful to look for evidence of conjunctival incisions, which can be helpful in determining whether previous surgery was performed on a particular muscle. Keep in mind that the incision may have been made at the limbus, in the fornix, or even over the muscle. One incision may have been used to approach more than one muscle.

Ductions and versions should be evaluated while looking particularly for underaction or overaction of previously operated muscles. Look for incomitance in different gaze positions and an inability to move the eye in the field of action of a particular muscle. In cases of overcorrection from an excessive recession, the forced duction or traction test will usually be negative. In overcorrections following an excessive resection, the forced duction test will often be positive, indicating a restriction. It may be easier and more reliable to perform forced duction testing with the patient under anesthesia.

In considering where to insert a previously operated muscle, it is essential to have committed to memory the "normal" average distances of the anatomic insertions of the muscles from the limbus (spiral of Tillaux) and to recall the orbital and fascial relationships of the extraocular muscles and tendons.

Case 1

ET = 60 got BMR recess = 6.5; now 2 months postop with ET = 30.

Surgeon 1: Resect the BLR 5 mm.

Surgeon 2: May wait 1 or 2 months, then resect the LR 8 mm OU if measurement unchanged.

Surgeon 3: Would wait; recheck fully atropinized cycloplegic refraction for evolving hyperopia, then rerecess the BMR 3 mm; right eye on adjustable suture, which allows for same-day adjustment under local anesthesia, as described in the discussion and references.[4]

Case 2

ET = 60 got BMR recess = 6.5; now 6 months postop with ET = 30.

Surgeon 1: Resect the LR 5 mm OU.

Surgeon 2: Resect the LR 8 mm OU.

Surgeon 3: Rerecess the BMR 3 mm; right eye on adjustable suture.[4]

Case 3

ET = 60 got BMR recess = 3; now 2 months postop with ET = 45.

Surgeon 1: Rerecess the BMR an additional 3.5 mm.

Surgeon 2: Rerecess the BMR an additional 2.5 mm.

Surgeon 3: Rerecess the BMR an additional 3.5 mm; right eye on a modified adjustable suture.

Case 4

ET = 50 got BMR recess = 6; now there is a consecutive XT = 20.

Surgeon 1: Advance MR of nondominant eye 4 mm (approximately 2 mm posterior to its original insertion).

Surgeon 2: Recess the LR 5 mm OU.

Surgeon 3: Explore both medial recti, which may have slipped. Advance both medial recti by 3 mm, putting one muscle on a modified adjustable suture.

Case 5

ET = 50 got BMR recess = 6; now 2 months postop with XT = 45.

Surgeon 1: I would be very concerned for a slipped muscle or a stretch scar. Carefully check ductions preoperatively. Explore both medial rectus muscles. If they both appeared healthy and in the expected position, I would advance both to close to their original insertion.

Surgeon 2: Advance the BMR 3 mm.

Surgeon 3: Explore both medial recti, which may have slipped. Advance both medial recti by 5 mm; put one muscle on a modified adjustable suture.

Case 6

ET = 30 got RMR recess = 4.5, RLR resect = 8; now 6 months postop with AET = 30.

Surgeon 1: Recess the LMR 4.5 mm and resect the LLR 5.5 mm.

Surgeon 2: Rerecess the RMR an additional 3 mm.

Surgeon 3: Recess the LMR 6.5 mm on modified adjustable suture.

Case 7

ET = 30 got RMR recess = 4.5, RLR resect = 8; now 9 months postop with XT = 20.

Surgeon 1: Recess the BLR 5 mm.
Surgeon 2: Recess the BLR 5 mm.
Surgeon 3: Recess the RLR 4.5 mm on modified adjustable suture.

Case 8

Sensory RXT = 40 got RMR resect = 6, RLR recess = 8; now 3 months postop with RXT = 40.

Surgeon 1: Rerecess the RLR 2 to 3 mm more and reresect the RMR 2 to 3 mm, being sure to check forced ductions so as not to create a significant restriction in abduction. Also RIO recession without myectomy 14 mm and RSO tenotomy to weaken all abducting forces.
Surgeon 2: Reresect the RMR 4 mm and rerecess the RLR 4 mm.
Surgeon 3: Reresect the RMR 3 mm and rerecess the RLR 4 mm.

Case 9

Three years after surgical correction for Case 8; now has RXT = 40.

Surgeon 1: Recess the LLR 7.5 mm and resect the LMR 6 mm.
Surgeon 2: Recess the LLR 8 mm and resect the LMR 6 mm.
Surgeon 3: Reresect the RMR 4 mm and RLR detachment with suturing to lateral orbital wall.

Case 10

Following surgery performed for Case 8, RET = 25 .

Surgeon 1: Recess the RMR 6 mm.
Surgeon 2: Recess the RMR 6 mm.
Surgeon 3: Recess the RMR 4 mm.

Case 11

XT = 25 got BLR recess = 6; now 2 months postop with XT = 25.

Surgeon 1: Resect the BMR 4.5 mm

Surgeon 2: May wait another 1 or 2 months, then resect the BMR 4.5 mm if stable.

Surgeon 3: Resect or plicate the BMR 4 mm.

Case 12

XT = 25 got BLR recess = 6; now 6 months postop with XT = 25.

Surgeon 1: Resect the BMR 4.5 mm.
Surgeon 2: Resect the BMR 4.5 mm.
Surgeon 3: Resect or plicate the BMR 4 mm.

Case 13

XT = 25 got BLR recess = 4; now 6 months postop with XT = 25.

Surgeon 1: Rerecess BLR an additional 4 mm.
Surgeon 2: Rerecess BLR 3 mm OU or resect BMR 4.5 mm.
Surgeon 3: Resect MR 4 mm in nondominant eye and rerecess the LR 3 mm on modified adjustable suture in the same eye.

Case 14

XT = 55 got BLR recess = 10; now 9 months postop with XT = 25.

Surgeon 1: Resect the BMR 5 mm.
Surgeon 2: Resect the BMR 4.5 mm.
Surgeon 3: Resect the BMR 3 mm.

Case 15

XT = 30 got BLR recess = 8 and RMR resect = 6; now 2 months postop with ET = 30.

Surgeon 1: Recess the BMR 4.5 mm.
Surgeon 2: EUA and forced ductions and plan to recess the RMR 6 mm; if forced ductions negative on attempted adduction, which indicates possible slipped or overrecessed lateral rectus muscle, would advance the RLR 8 mm and recess the RMR 4 mm.
Surgeon 3: Recess the RMR 5 mm on modified adjustable suture.

Case 16

XT = 20 got RLR recess = 8; now 6 months postop with XT = 20.

Surgeon 1: Recess the LLR 8 mm.
Surgeon 2: Resect the BMR 4.5 mm.
Surgeon 3: Recess the LLR 3 mm on modified adjustable suture.

Case 17

XT = 20 got RLR recess = 11; now 6 months postop with XT = 20.

Surgeon 1: Recess the LLR 8 mm.
Surgeon 2: Resect the BMR 4.5 mm.
Surgeon 3: Recess the LLR 5 mm on modified adjustable suture.

Case 18

XT = 20 got RLR recess = 9; now 2 years postop with ET = 20.

Surgeon 1: Advance the RLR to close to its original insertion.
Surgeon 2: Advance the RLR 4.5 mm.
Surgeon 3: Explore and advance the RLR 4 mm.

Case 19

XT = 35 got RLR recess = 8, resect RMR = 6; now 2 months postop with XT = 25.

Surgeon 1: Recess the LLR 9 mm.
Surgeon 2: With negative intraoperative forced duction testing, resect the LMR 7 mm. If forced duction positive on adduction, recess the LLR 6 mm and resect the LMR 5 mm.
Surgeon 3: Recess the LLR 5 mm and resect the LMR 4 mm.

Case 20

XT = 35 got RLR recess = 8, RMR resect = 6; now 2 months postop with ET = 35.

Surgeon 1: Recess the BMR 5 mm.
Surgeon 2: Forced ductions and probably recess the RMR 4.5 mm or asymmetrically recess the MR OU OD > OS.
Surgeon 3: Recess the RMR 5 mm.

Case 21

Status post-recess RMR and resect RLR OD for ET then recess LMR and resect LLR OS for ET; now 2 years postop with XT = 40.

Surgeon 1: Recess the BLR 8 mm.
Surgeon 2: Recess the BLR 7 mm.
Surgeon 3: Recess the BLR 6 mm.

Case 22

ET = 50 got BMR recess = 6, then went XT = 30 got BLR recess = 7; now 6 months postop with ET = 30.

Surgeon 1: Advance one LR to close to its original insertion, reevaluate in 2 months, and consider advancing the other LR if needed.
Surgeon 2: Advance the BLR 4 mm.
Surgeon 3: Advance the BLR 3.5 mm.

Case 23

XT' > XT got BMR resect = 5; now 2 months postop with ET = 30.

Surgeon 1: Recess the BMR 4.5 mm.
Surgeon 2: Recess the BMR 3.5 mm.
Surgeon 3: Recess the BMR 3 mm.

Discussion

In formulating a surgical plan for strabismus reoperation, one must first consider why the previous untoward results may have occurred in the face of reasonable surgical numbers. The interaction of variable or inaccurate preoperative measurements, muscle malposition (eg, excessive recessions or resections) or slippage, and scar formation must be considered. Violation of Tenon's capsule with fat prolapse, termed *adherence syndrome*, may result in scar formation between the muscle and the globe, which will likely restrict motility.[5] Some of these causes will be discovered only during surgery with direct observation, but preoperative traction or forced duction testing can help guide the surgeon to the more likely area of concern. In other cases, no explanation for an overcorrection or undercorrection will be recognized. In all cases, the previous surgery, present measurements and motility, and intraoperative findings must be considered before formulating an optimal surgical approach.

Cases 1 and 2 involve undercorrections following a large BMR recession (6.5 mm) for an ET of 60, the only difference being the time following surgery (2 vs 6 months). Some would observe for more than 2 months before surgical intervention, perhaps because the deviation could change or vary but also because it is difficult for some patients or parents to accept further surgery so soon. An additional consideration is the age of the patient. If a child is younger than 24 months, earlier surgery might be considered to salvage limited binocularity, as in the monofixation syndrome.[6] Bilateral lateral rectus muscle resection is a popular option. The amount to resect each lateral rectus muscle is based on individual experience and/or surgical dosing tables (eg, I would use 7-mm resections for an XT of 30). A decision to do less of a resection may be appropriate if there is some underaction of the previously recessed medial rectus muscles. Another option is to rerecess the medial rectus muscles. Recessions greater than 6.5 mm may result in an adduction deficit, which could result in progressive exotropia. One surgeon chose to perform rerecessions using a modified adjustable suture on one of the medial rectus muscles. This technique involves recessing the muscle using an adjustable suture that can be left without tying when the patient is awake or that can be adjusted within a few hours after surgery following sedation or the readministration of general anesthesia.[4] As in many cases, an adjustable suture allows the surgeon to determine the alignment on the day of surgery. The disadvantage is that additional anesthesia with intervention on the day of the initial surgery may be required, especially in children.

Case 3 involves a large-angle esotropia for which a smaller BMR recession of 3 mm was done and significant undercorrection resulted. A rerecession of the medial rectus muscles is a good option and is less likely to produce an adduction deficit. Another option is to rerecess the medial rectus muscle and resect one lateral rectus muscle in the nonfixating eye, depending on how many millimeters of MR recession one is comfortable in performing.

Surgery for consecutive exotropia following a BMR recession for ET, as in Cases 4 and 5, should be planned on the basis of the amount of the initial medial rectus recession and the amount of underaction of the operated medial rectus muscles. In Case 4, an XT of 20 resulted. One option is to perform a BLR recession. Surgeons concerned that the overcorrection may be related to excessive weakening of one or both medial rectus muscles could elect to explore either medial rectus muscle depending on which seems to be underacting or in the nonfixating eye. The muscle can then be advanced. The surgical decision to explore and advance the medial rectus muscles becomes unanimous following a larger (XT = 40) overcorrection. It is most likely that adduction deficits will be recognized on evaluation of the patient's ductions, which will make the decision easier. Once again, one surgeon would use a modified adjustable suture on one of the medial muscles. However, it is more difficult to increase the amount of recession during the adjustment than to reduce it.

The approach to an undercorrection of an ET following a unilateral recess/resect procedure, as in Case 6, would lead some surgeons to perform a similar procedure on the opposite eye by using only a medial rectus recession for the lesser amount of correction needed. An additional recession of the previously recessed medial rectus muscle with or without an adjustable suture is an option. It may be difficult to correct an ET of 40, however, without a large medial rectus muscle recession, which could produce an adduction deficit.

In Case 7, a small-to-moderate consecutive XT following a unilateral recession/resection for an ET is most easily approached by recessing one or both lateral rectus muscles. Patients with sensory XT are less likely to have stable results because of the absence of binocularity and fusional vergences. It may be preferred to leave the eye with the reduced vision slightly ET unless there is a highly hyperopic refractive error in the fixating eye.

In Case 8, after a recess/resect procedure for an RXT of 40, the patient was left with an XT of 40. All 3 surgeons suggest resecting the medial rectus an additional 3 to 4 mm and recessing the lateral rectus muscle an additional 4 mm. One surgeon suggests weakening both oblique muscles in the exotropic eye to weaken all abducting forces. This is an original approach that may help as long as the vertical forces are balanced. In the absence of binocularity, postoperative torsional diplopia would not be likely to occur.

As often occurs in patients with sensory exotropia, the patient in Case 9 reverted to an XT of 40. Now a careful explanation of why one would elect to operate on the normally seeing eye is in order and a recess/resect procedure on the left eye may be performed. A nonconventional solution would be to detach the right lateral rectus muscle and suture it to the lateral orbital wall, which would negate its effect yet leave it retrievable. At the same time, the right medial rectus muscle could be resected again. These solutions might result in a consecutive esotropia, as in Case 10. A 4- to 6-mm resection of the right medial rectus muscle is suggested. An adjustable suture would help to ensure a preferred position in the immediate postoperative period.

In Case 11, after a BLR recession of 6 for an XT of 25, there is a residual XT of 25 at 2 months postoperatively. All three surgeons suggest resecting the medial rectus muscles in both eyes 4.5 to 6 mm, one after observing the patient for another month for stability of measurements. In Case 12, at 6 months after surgery, very similar recommendations are made. In Case 13, there was a residual XT of 25 following recessions of only 4 mm of each lateral rectus muscle. This would be expected to be insufficient, and 2 of the surgeons would recess each lateral rectus muscle an additional 3 or 4 mm. Other options include adding a medial rectus resection in both eyes or in one eye coupled with an additional recession of one lateral rectus muscle. How much of an effect can be expected from a large BLR recession? In Case 14, a residual XT of 25 following a BLR recession of 10 mm for an XT of 55 is seen. In this case, a resection of both medial rectus muscles of 3 to 5 mm is suggested as a solution. Distance/near disparity in the XT must be considered. For larger exodeviations, a BLR recession may not be as effective; if you have a basic type in which the XT at near fixation is the same as at distance fixation, a medial rectus resection is usually added. This was done in Case 15, in which an overcorrection of an ET of 30 resulted. Suggestions to correct this consecutive ET include recessing the previously resected medial rectus muscle 5 to 6 mm or a BMR recession of 4.5 mm.

Unilateral LR recessions are useful in correcting lesser amounts of exotropia, especially if there is a divergence excess type. In Case 16, the RLR was recessed 8 mm for an XT of 20 with no improvement in alignment. To correct this, the LLR could be recessed 8 mm, or if the deviation was present at near fixation, the LMR could be resected 4.5 mm each.

In Case 17, the RLR was recessed 11 mm to correct an XT of 20, and no correction was achieved. Once again, the opposite lateral rectus muscle could be recessed or the medial rectus resected in one or both eyes. The deviation at near fixation must be considered to avoid an overcorrection.

In Case 18, following a recession of the RLR 9 mm for an XT of 20, a consecutive ET of 20 results. This is an unexpected result and indicates a possible slipped lateral rectus muscle. An advancement of the previously operated lateral rectus muscle of 4, 5, or even 8 mm, depending on where it is found during surgery, is a good choice.

In Case 19, to correct an XT of 35, the RLR is recessed 8 mm and the RMR is resected 6 mm, leading to a residual XT of 25. The preference in this case is to operate on the left eye unless there is a limitation of adduction, in which case the left medial rectus muscle should be explored. Solutions include recessing the LLR 9 mm, recessing the LLR 5 or 6 mm coupled with resecting the LMR 4 or 5 mm, or simply resecting the LMR 7 mm.

The same initial surgery performed in Case 19 results in an ET of 35 in Case 20. In a reversal of this magnitude, a slipped lateral rectus is suspected, particularly if there is limited abduction. This consecutive ET might best be managed with an RMR recession of 4.5 to 5 mm or a BMR recession of 5 mm.

In Case 21, a consecutive XT of 40 results following recessions of the RMR and LMR and resections of the RLR and LLR for an ET of undetermined magnitude. Solutions include BLR recession of 6 to 8 mm. The amount of recession might be determined by the location of the previously resected lateral rectus muscle and the amount of restriction found intraoperatively. For an ET of 50, a BMR recession of 6 leads to an XT of 30 in Case 22. A BLR of 7 then results in an ET of 30. Reasonable options in this case include advancing both LR 3.5 or 4 mm or advancing one LR to the original insertion. On average, the original anatomic insertion of the lateral rectus should be located about 6.9 mm from the limbus. This is important to know because in some reoperations, the anatomic insertion may be unrecognizable and you can recreate it by measuring with a caliper.

Finally, Case 23 illustrates the difficulty in surgically managing patients with XT with convergence insufficiency. This patient underwent resections of both medial rectus muscles for 5 mm. An ET of 30 resulted, and the patient most likely would have experienced diplopia if he or she were an adult. The suggested solution is a BMR recession of 3 to 5 mm. If there were a distance/near disparity in the ET, the decision as to what surgery to perform would be more difficult. Considering that some pediatric ophthalmologists believe that the medial rectus muscle might be more effective at near fixation while the lateral rectus muscle is more effective at distance fixation, should be included in surgical planning.

Managing a reoperation requires careful preoperative planning. Knowledge of the previous surgical procedure or procedures is helpful but cannot always be relied on. The strabismus surgeon must be prepared to handle unexpected intraoperative findings to achieve optimal results.

REFERENCES

1. Cooper EL. The surgical management of secondary exotropia. *Trans Am Acad Ophthalmol Otolaryngol.* 1961;65:595.
2. Sirvastava SK, Reichman OS, Lambert SR. The use of an image guidance system in retrieving lost medial rectus muscles. *J AAPOS.* 2002;6(5):309-314.
3. Demer JL, Clark RA, Kono R, et al. A 12-year, prospective study of extraocular muscle imaging in complex strabismus. *J AAPOS.* 2002;6(6):337-347.
4. Engel EM, Rousta ST. Adjustable sutures in children using a modified technique. *J AAPOS.* 2004;8(3):243-248.
5. Parks MM. The overacting inferior oblique muscle. *Am J Ophthalmol.* 1974;77:787.
6. Ing MR. Early surgical alignment for congenital esotropia. *Trans Am Ophthalmol Soc.* 1981;79:625-663.

10

Nystagmus

Leonard B. Nelson, MD, MBA

Nystagmus is a condition of involuntary repetitive eye movements; it can occur in infancy or later in life and is often associated with decreased visual acuity. The field of gaze in which the nystagmus intensity is absent or least is termed the *null position*. If the null position is fortuitously located in the primary position, there is no need for a compensatory head posture. However, a null point may be located in lateral gaze to either side or less commonly in elevation, depression, or obliquely. When a patient has such an eccentric null position, he or she will assume an anomalous head posture to maximize visual acuity, dampening the nystagmus by placing the eyes in the field of gaze. This allows the patient to look straight ahead with the eyes in the position of gaze, which corresponds to the null position. Strabismus, especially esotropia, and significant refractive error are commonly associated with nystagmus.

There are several steps in the clinical evaluation that will assist in the decision-making process for surgery in patients with nystagmus. Accurate correction of any significant refractive error should be instituted in an attempt to improve vision and visual function. Abnormal head posture can be evaluated and measured by having the patient fixate on the smallest possible target at distance. The anomalous head position becomes more prominent with increasing visual demand. In some patients, it will be necessary to include additional testing—such as neuroimaging, neurologic testing, and eletrophysiologic recordings—to elucidate the cause of low vision and nystagmus. If there is an underlying disorder, the ophthalmologist should consider whether

Nelson LB, Levin AV, eds.
The Wills Eye Strabismus Surgery Handbook (pp 99-104).
© 2015 Taylor & Francis Group.

there is an intervention (eg, cataract surgery) that could improve vision before considering nystagmus surgery. It is also important to measure the vision while fogging the untested eye to avoid additional blurring, which will occur if latent nystagmus is stimulated by complete occlusion of the eye not being tested. Binocular distance and near visual acuity should also be recorded while the child is allowed to assume the head position.

If it is determined that no further medical therapy will improve the ocular motion abnormality, eye muscle surgery may be indicated. There are a number of possible indications for eye muscle surgery in patients with nystagmus. If a patient with nystagmus has a significant anomalous head posture, eye muscle surgery can move the null position to the primary position. In patients with strabismus, eye muscle surgery can reduce the strabismus and improve any associated anomalous head posture. Obtaining some degree of fusion may also help to dampen the nystagmus. Finally, in patients with nystagmus without an anomalous head posture or strabismus, eye muscle surgery may reduce nystagmus intensity and improve visual acuity.

Case 1

A 4-year-old boy with oculocutaneous albinism and horizontal symmetric nystagmus, 20/200 each eye, no face turn or strabismus.

Surgeon 1: No surgery.

Surgeon 2: Observation or tenotomy of all 4 horizontal recti and reattachment.

Surgeon 3: Tenotomy of all 4 horizontal recti and reattachment.

Case 2

20/200 OD and 20/30 OS from right more than left optic nerve hypoplasia. RET = 45. Left face turn = 25 degrees, horizontal nystagmus.

Surgeon 1: Recess the LMR 6 mm on hang back and recess the RMR 5 mm adjustable. If family refuses surgery on OS, then recess the RMR 6 mm adjustable and resect the RLR 5 mm.

Surgeon 2: OS is driving face turn. Recess the LMR 6 mm and resect the LLR 8 mm.

Surgeon 3: Recess the BMR 5 mm.

Case 3

Same patient as Case 2 except RXT = 45.

Surgeon 1: Recess the RLR 8 mm and resect the RMR 5 mm.

Surgeon 2: Recess the RLR 9 mm and resect the RMR 7 mm.

Surgeon 3: Resect the RMR 5 mm, recess the LMR 6 mm, and resect the LLR 7 mm.

Case 4

20/40 OU. Chin down = 25 degrees. No strabismus, horizontal symmetric nystagmus.

Surgeon 1: Recess the BSR 5 mm and recess the BIO 14 mm.

Surgeon 2: Recess the BSR 7 mm.

Surgeon 3: Recess the BSR 5 mm and resect the BIR 5 mm.

Case 5

Same patient as Case 4 except chin up = 25 degrees.

Surgeon 1: Recess the BIO 14 mm without myectomy and recess the SR 6 mm.

Surgeon 2: Undercorrect as downgaze needed. Recess the BIR 5.5 mm.

Surgeon 3: Resect the BSR 5 mm and recess the BIR 5 mm.

Case 6

Horizontal nystagmus, right face turn = 25 degrees. No strabismus. VA 20/80 OU.

Surgeon 1: Recess the LLR 10.5 mm and recess the RMR 7.5 mm, both on adjustable sutures.

Surgeon 2: Kestenbaum +40% augmented: recess the RMR 7 mm, resect the LMR 8.5 mm, recess the LLR 10 mm, and resect the RLR 11 mm.

Surgeon 3: Recess RMR 6 mm, resect RLR 8 mm, resect LMR 6 mm, recess LLR 9 mm.

Case 7

A 5-year-old child enucleated for unilateral retinoblastoma OD.

VA OS 20/30, left face turn = 25 degrees with horizontal pendular nystagmus OS.

Surgeon 1: Recess the LMR 6.5-mm hang back.

Surgeon 2: Resect the LLR 10 mm and recess the LMR 6.5 mm.

Surgeon 3: Recess the LMR 4 mm and resect the LLR 5 mm.

Discussion

Prior to 2000, there was no surgical treatment for patients with nystagmus who did not have associated strabismus or anomalous head position and null position.[1] Recently, the 4-muscle tenotomy procedure, which involves detaching and immediately reattaching the 2 horizontal rectus muscles in each eye to their original insertions, has shown positive therapeutic effects. These results have been documented by extensive eye movement recordings showing lengthening foveation time and reducing nystagmus intensity.[1] As a result of the 4-muscle tenotomy procedure, there is a generalized broadening of the null position and an improvement in central vision in many of these patients. As illustrated by the responses in Case 1, it is presently an accepted treatment option for patients with nystagmus without strabismus or an anomalous head posture and is being performed by a number of pediatric ophthalmologists throughout the United States and worldwide. Studies beyond the use of eye movement recordings will hopefully further elucidate the clinical benefits of this procedure.

Patients with nystagmus and a compensatory horizontal head posture without strabismus (Case 6) can benefit from eye muscle surgery that shifts the null gaze from an eccentric position to the primary position. The most popular surgical procedure for the correction of an abnormal head position in patients with nystagmus is a modification of the operations initially described by Anderson and Kestenbaum.[1] The modification that is most commonly accepted by pediatric ophthalmologists is that proposed by Parks.[2] He advocated horizontal rectus muscle surgery of 5, 6, 7, and 8 mm with a total of 13 mm of surgery performed on each eye. Surgery of 5 and 6 mm was always performed on the medial rectus muscles, the former with a recession and the latter with a resection. Surgery of 7 and 8 mm was performed on the lateral rectus muscles, again the former with a recession and the latter with a resection. A recession of the medial rectus of the adducted eye is combined with a resection of the ipsilateral lateral rectus; a resection of the medial rectus of the abducted eye is combined with a recession of the ipsilateral lateral rectus. Parks believed, at the time of his recommendation, that the amount of surgery he proposed was the maximum that could be performed to preserve full ductions.[2]

Because of the high rate of residual face turn in patients using Parks' guidelines, an augmented modified Kestenbaum procedure has been proposed.[3] Adding 40% to each muscle's surgery for face turns of 25 degrees and 60% for larger face turns has resulted in a more sustained surgical correction for the abnormal head position. Preoperatively, these patients essentially have a gaze palsy in the direction of the head turn where their nystagmus intensity is greatest. Postoperatively, a gaze palsy is created in the opposite direction. In my experience, parents and patients prefer the more normal head position and do not complain about the decreased field of rotation. Another modification of the Kestenbaum procedure was proposed by von Noorden[4] and involves a lateral rectus recession of the abducted eye and a medial rectus recession of the adducted eye. One potential advantage of this procedure is that it leaves 2 horizontal muscles unoperated in patients who may have both a horizontal and vertical head posture. Therefore, surgery can be performed on both the horizontal and vertical muscles without concern about the risk of anterior segment ischemia. The results of this modification still require further study.

In patients with nystagmus, abnormal head posture, and strabismus, the position of the head is determined by the preferred position of gaze of the fixating eye. In cases 2 and 3, the left eye with the 20/30 vision is the preferred or fixating eye. Any change in the head position will be mediated by the fixating eye. Therefore, surgery performed on the fixating eye will eliminate or improve the abnormal head posture. Additional surgery on the nonfixating eye will be necessary for residual strabismus. This may be accomplished either at the time of surgery on the fixating eye or as a subsequent operation. For patients with esotropia, nystagmus, and an abnormal face turn (Case 2), it may be possible to correct the face turn and strabismus by just operating on the fixating eye. By correcting the face turn, the amount of surgery on the preferred eye may be enough so that no further surgery will be necessary on the nonfixating eye. In patients with exotropia (Case 3), operating on the preferred eye to correct the face turn will increase the exotropia. There are 2 basic approaches to the exotropic patient: (1) perform staged surgery, correcting the face turn by operating on the preferred eye and then attempting to correct the strabismus at a subsequent surgery, or (2) do simultaneous surgery and determine how much additional exotropia is induced by operating on the preferred eye and either perform only a large recession of the contralateral rectus or combine a lateral rectus recession of the medial rectus of the contralateral eye. Some pediatric ophthalmologists perform simultaneous surgery utilizing adjustable sutures to assist in obtaining the desired postoperative alignment.

Vertical head postures with nystagmus, either chin up (Case 5) or chin down (Case 4), are less common than horizontal face turns. Moderate (5 to 6 mm) to large (8 mm) vertical rectus muscle surgery is often necessary to correct vertical head position associated with nystagmus. I usually perform 8-mm bilateral superior rectus recession for chin-down patients (Case 4) and 8-mm bilateral inferior rectus recession for patients with chin up of 25 degrees. If further surgery is necessary, resections on the opposite vertical rectus muscles can be done. Simultaneous moderate-to-large amounts of surgery on the vertical rectus muscles have been successful in correcting the vertical head postures as well. Vertical head posture and nystagmus have also been treated with success by operating on the oblique muscles. For the chin-down position (Case 4), moderate bilateral superior rectus recessions combined with bilateral inferior oblique recessions have been successful. Both elevators are weakened, with a reduction in the chin-down position. Conversely, for a chin-up position, bilateral superior oblique tenotomy or tenectomy combined with a bilateral moderate inferior rectus recession reduces the effect of the depressors and improves the vertical head position. Because of the rarity of chin-up and chin-down positions with nystagmus and the lack of consensus on the appropriate treatment, further studies are necessary.

Infantile monocular blindness may result in bilateral nystagmus.[5] This may occur as well with monocular enucleation in early childhood (Case 7).[6] It is thought that the blind eye acts essentially as an occluder, allowing latent nystagmus to become manifest.[6] The nystagmus is then in adduction, resulting in a face turn toward the "normal" eye. The goal of surgery is to move the null point from adduction to the primary position. For face turns of 25 degrees, a recession of the medial rectus and resection of the lateral rectus in the fixating eye will be necessary to correct the face turn. Usually, a large medial rectus recession and lateral rectus resection are used. This procedure will require a detailed discussion and explanation to parents, who may feel quite uncomfortable in contemplating surgery on their child's only "good" eye.

REFERENCES

1. Hertle RW, Dell'Osso LF. *Nystagmus in Infancy and Childhood*. New York, NY: Oxford University Press; 2013.
2. Parks MM. Congenital nystagmus surgery. *Am Ophthalmol J*. 1973;23:35-39.
3. Nelson LB, Ervin-Mulvey LD, Calhoun JH, Harley RD, Keisler MS. Surgical management for abnormal head position in nystagmus: the augmented modified Kestenbaum procedure. *Br J Ophthalmol*. 1984;68:796-800.
4. Von Noorden GK. *Binocular Vision and Ocular Motility: Theory and Management of Strabismus*. 5th ed. St. Louis, MO: Mosby-Yearbook; 1996.
5. Kushner BJ. Infantile uniocular blindness with bilateral nystagmus: a syndrome. *Arch Ophthalmol*. 1995;113:1296-1300.
6. Helveston EM, Pinchoff B, Ellis FD, Miller K. Unilateral esotropia after enucleation in infancy. *Am J Ophthalmol*. 1985;100:96-99.

FINANCIAL DISCLOSURES

Dr. Miles J. Burke has no financial or proprietary interest in the materials presented herein.

Dr. Kammi Gunton has no financial or proprietary interest in the materials presented herein.

Dr. Stephen P. Kraft has no financial or proprietary interest in the materials presented herein.

Dr. Alex V. Levin has reported no financial or proprietary interest in the materials presented herein.

Dr. Leonard B. Nelson has no financial or proprietary interest in the materials presented herein.

Dr. Mary O'Hara has no financial or proprietary interest in the materials presented herein.

Dr. Scott Olitsky has no financial or proprietary interest in the materials presented herein.

Dr. Sepideh Tara Rousta has no financial or proprietary interest in the materials presented herein.

Dr. Mark A. Steele has no financial or proprietary interest in the materials presented herein.

Dr. Rudolph S. Wagner has no financial or proprietary interest in the materials presented herein.

Dr. Daniel T. Weaver has no financial or proprietary interest in the materials presented herein.

INDEX

acrocephalosyndactyly (Apert syndrome), 58, 64–65

adherence syndrome, 93

adjustable sutures, 22–23, 34–35, 40, 57–58, 60–62, 76, 79, 83, 87–92, 94–95, 101, 103

albinism, oculocutaneous, 100

alternating esotropia, 77, 78, 89–90. *See also* cyclic esotropia

alternating exotropia, 23, 60, 67

amblyopia
    complex cases, 80–82
    dissociated vertical deviation and, 27
    esotropia and, 9–10, 13
    exotropia and, 18, 21–22
    surgical decision making, 3, 4
    systemic diseases and, 63–66
    third-nerve palsy and, 35

aneurysm, 38

anomalous retinal correspondence (ARC), 16, 22

anterior plagiocephaly, 59, 63–64, 66

anterior transposition of the inferior oblique, 27–31

A-patterns, 16, 65, 70

Apert syndrome, 58, 64–65

aphakia, 76–77, 81–82

ARC (anomalous retinal correspondence), 16, 22

Arnold-Chiari malformation, 60, 70

botulinum toxin, 33–34, 39, 41, 42

brain tumor, 39

Brown syndrome, 48, 51–52, 83

cataract surgery, 80–81

cerebral palsy, 60, 67

CFEOM (congenital fibrosis of the extraocular muscles), 48–49, 53

comitance, spread of, 41

complex strabismus cases, 75–86

congenital cranial dysinnervation disorders, 49–51

congenital esotropia, 8, 12, 31

congenital exotropia, 16–17, 20, 31

congenital fibrosis of the extraocular muscles (CFEOM), 48–49, 53

congenital fourth-nerve palsy, 36

congenital glaucoma, 83

congenital third-nerve palsy, 35–36, 40

convergence insufficiency exotropia, 15, 18–19, 22

Cooper's law, 87

corneal transplants, 80, 83–84

cranial nerve palsies, 33–43
    acute-onset, 33–34
    Arnold-Chiari malformation and, 70
    fourth-nerve, 36–38, 41, 64
    sixth-nerve, 3, 33–34, 38–39, 41–42, 47, 49, 50
    strabismus syndromes and, 47, 49, 50
    third-nerve, 34–36, 40, 49

craniosynostosis, 58–59, 63–66

cyclic esotropia, 47, 51

Dandy-Walker malformation, 70

DEP (double elevator palsy), 47, 52–53

diplopia, 2
    complex strabismus cases, 77, 78, 79–81, 83
    cranial nerve palsies, 3, 38, 42
    postoperative
        congenital fibrosis and, 53
        exotropia, surgery for, 16, 19, 22, 23–24
        thyroid orbitopathy, 62
    preoperative testing, 81
    systemic diseases, 60, 61, 69–70, 71

dissociated strabismus complex, 25
dissociated vertical deviation (DVD), 12, 25–32, 64
divergence excess exotropia, 15, 19, 22
double elevator palsy (DEP), 47, 52–53
Down syndrome, 59, 66–67
Duane retraction syndrome (DRS), 3, 46, 49–50
DVD (dissociated vertical deviation), 12, 25–32, 64

enucleation, monocular, 101, 104
esotropia
    common cases and discussion, 7–14
    complex cases, 76–77, 78, 80, 84–85
    dissociated vertical deviation and, 12, 31
    nystagmus and, 99, 100, 103
    preoperative counseling, 3
    reoperations, 14, 88–97
    sixth-nerve palsy, 3, 38–39, 41–42
    strabismus syndromes, 46, 47, 49, 50–51
    systemic diseases, 58, 59, 60, 61, 62–63, 66, 69–71
esotropia, cyclic, 47, 51
esotropia, mixed-mechanism, 13–14
exophoria, 15
exotropia
    common cases and discussion, 15–24
    complex strabismus cases, 77, 78, 79, 80–81
    dissociated vertical deviation and, 28, 31
    nystagmus and, 100–101, 103
    reoperations, 20, 21, 23–24, 89–97
    strabismus syndromes, 46, 49, 51
    systemic diseases, 59, 60, 64, 65–66, 67, 68
    third-nerve palsy and, 34–36, 40

Faden operation, 13, 30–31
force duction/forced generation testing, 40, 42
fourth-nerve palsy, 36–38, 41, 64
Fresnel lenses, 16, 22, 23

gaze palsy, 102–103
glaucoma surgery, 78, 80, 83

Harada-Ito procedure, 37–38, 41
head posture, anomalous, 2, 45, 64, 99, 100–104
Hummelsheim procedure, 84
hydrocephalus, 70
hyperopia
    complex strabismus cases, 78, 82, 84–85
    dissociated vertical deviation and, 28
    Duane retraction syndrome, 49
    esotropia and, 10–11, 13–14
    exotropia and, 20, 23
    nystagmus and, 99
    systemic diseases, 59, 66
hypertropia
    complex strabismus cases, 78–79, 80
    cranial nerve palsies, 34, 36–38, 40, 41
    vs dissociated vertical deviation, 26
    systemic diseases, 59, 64
hypotropia
    strabismus syndromes, 47, 48–49, 51–53
    systemic diseases, 57, 58–59, 62, 65–66
    third-nerve palsy and, 35–36, 40

incomitance in exotropia, lateral, 16, 19–20, 23
infantile esotropia, 8, 12, 31
infantile exotropia, 16–17, 20, 31
infantile monocular blindness, 101, 104
inferior oblique, anterior transposition of, 27–31
inferior oblique palsy, 51
intermittent exotropia, 15–16, 67
intermittent hypotropia, 35–36
internuclear ophthalmoplegia, 60, 68

Jensen procedure, 41, 50–51, 84

Kestenbaum procedure, 102–103
Knapp procedure, 47, 52–53, 58, 79, 84

large-angle esotropia, 12
large-angle exotropia, 20
LASIK/LASEK surgery, 78, 84–85
lateral incomitance in exotropia, 16, 19–20, 23
lateral rectus palsy, 83
lost or slipped rectus muscle, 78–79, 84, 89

microphthalmia, aphakia with, 76–77, 82
Möbius syndrome, 47, 50–51
monocular elevation deficiency, 52–53
"morning glory" syndrome, 80, 81–82
multiple sclerosis, 60, 67–68
myasthenia gravis, 60, 68–70
myopia, 20, 82

null position, 99, 100, 102
nystagmus, 25–26, 99–104

oculocutaneous albinism, 100
ophthalmoplegia, internuclear, 60, 68
optic atrophy, 63
optic nerve hypoplasia, 100–101

Parkinson's disease, 61, 71
Parks' guidelines, 102
patch test, 15
patient, preoperative consultation with, 3–4
patient history and examination, 1
persistent fetal vasculature, 76, 81–82
plagiocephaly, 59, 63–64, 66
posterior fixation suture, 13, 30–31
posterior plagiocephaly, 63–64
postoperative adjustments. *See* reoperations
postoperative diplopia, 16, 19, 22, 23–24, 53, 62
prism spectacles, 16, 22, 23
proptosis, 61
pseudoptosis, 47, 52
pterygium surgery, 79
ptosis, 35–36, 40, 52, 53, 69

recession vs resection procedures, 4–5
rectus muscle, slipped or lost, 78–79, 84, 89

red lens testing, 22, 81
refractive surgery, strabismus after, 78, 84–85
reoperations
    Brown syndrome, 51–52
    cases and discussion, 87–97
    esotropia, 14, 88–97
    exotropia, 20, 21, 23–24, 89–97
    thyroid orbitopathy, 62
resection vs recession procedures, 4–5
retinal detachment surgery, 77, 82–83
retinoblastoma, enucleation for, 101, 104

scar formation, 48, 52, 75, 83, 93
scleral buckle, 77, 82–83
sensory exotropia, 90, 95
seventh-nerve palsy, 47, 50
silicone expanders, 48, 52
sixth-nerve palsy
    acute-onset, 33–34
    cases, 38–39
    discussion, 41–42
    preoperative counseling, 3
    strabismus syndromes, 47, 49, 50
slipped or lost rectus muscle, 78–79, 84, 89
small-angle exotropia, 20
socially acceptable alignment, 76, 81–82
strabismus surgery, decision-making approach to, 1–5
    history and examination, 1
    patient, discussion with, 3–4
    surgical approach, development of, 4–5
    treatment objectives, 2
strabismus surgery reoperations. *See* reoperations
strabismus syndromes, 45–55
    Brown syndrome, 48, 51–52, 83
    congenital fibrosis, 48–49, 53
    cyclic esotropia, 47, 51
    double elevator palsy, 47, 52–53
    Duane retraction syndrome, 3, 46, 49–50
    Möbius syndrome, 47, 50–51
superior oblique palsy, 21, 64, 66, 83
superior temporal trabeculectomy, 78

suppression scotomas, 76, 81
surgery reoperations, 87–97
systemic disease, strabismus in, 57–73
    Arnold-Chiari malformation, 60, 70
    cerebral palsy, 60, 67
    craniosynostosis, 58–59, 63–66
    Down syndrome, 59, 66–67
    multiple sclerosis, 60, 67–68
    myasthenia gravis, 60, 68–70
    Parkinson's disease, 61, 71
    thyroid orbitopathy, 57–58, 61–63

tendon suture spacers, 52
third-nerve palsy, 34–36, 40, 49
thyroid orbitopathy, 57–58, 61–63
torsion, 33, 37–38, 41, 53, 64, 66, 82–83
torticollis, 64, 70
trabeculectomy, 78

transposition procedures, 84
trauma, cranial nerve palsies and, 37–39,
    41, 42
traumatic transection of inferior rectus
    muscle, 78–79, 84

ultrasound biomicroscopy, 82

V-patterns
    Arnold-Chiari malformation, 70
    craniosynostosis, 64–65
    in esotropia, 8–9, 12–13, 77
    in exotropia, 16, 17–18, 20–21

Worth 4-dot testing, 81

Z tenotomy, 52

Printed in the United States
by Baker & Taylor Publisher Services